The Testosterone Solution

The Testosterone Solution

Increase Your Energy and Vigor with Male Hormone Therapy

AUBREY HILL, M.D.

Prima Publishing

PRIMA PUBLISHING and colophon are registered trademarks of Prima Communications, Inc.

Library of Congress Cataloging-in-Publication Data

Hill, Aubrey M.
The testosterone solution: increase your energy and vigor
with male hormone therapy / Aubrey Hill.
p. cm.
Includes bibliographical references and index.
ISBN 0-7615-1022-2
1.Testosterone—Therapeutic use. I. Title.
RM296.5 T47H54 1997
615' .366—DC21   97-13864
CIP
97 98 99 00 01 HH 10 9 8 7 6 5 4 3 2 1
Printed in the United States of America

Warning—Disclaimer
The information provided in this book is not intended to be a substitute for professional or medical advice. The author and publisher specifically disclaim any liability, loss or risk, personal or otherwise, which is incurred as a result, directly or indirectly, of the use and application of any of the contents of this book.

All products mentioned in this book are trademarks of their respective companies.

How to Order
Single copies may be ordered from Prima Publishing, P.O. Box 1260BK, Rocklin, CA 95677; telephone (916) 632-4400. Quantity discounts are also available. On your letterhead, include information concerning the intended use of the books and the number of books you wish to purchase.

Visit us online at www.primapublishing.com

*To the memory of Carl Heller, M.D., professor at the
University of Oregon Medical School,
the first person to arouse my interest in endocrinology*

CONTENTS

Contents

ACKNOWLEDGMENTS

I wish to acknowledge and thank the following people: Esther Hill, my wife and computer consultant, who gave me much encouragement, offered helpful comments and suggestions, and transmitted the manuscript via the Internet; Helen Clough, who typed the manuscript; Natasha Kern, literary agent, who very early believed in the project; Alice Price Knight, Professional Writing Services in Denver, who took my original manuscript, reorganized the chapters, and rewrote it so it would be comprehensible to the laity and of interest to a publisher; and Eric Orwoll, M.D., Oregon Health Sciences University and Elizabeth Barrett-Connor, M.D., School of Medicine, University of California, San Diego, whose expertise was useful in collecting the information needed in researching material for the book. I would also like to thank Laura Connor, R.N., for her reorganization of the manuscript and editorial revisions on several chapters.

INTRODUCTION

In my medical practice, I am constantly amazed at how little men know about their male anatomy and physiology or about their own sexuality. As men enter middle age, they may experience a decrease in their sexual prowess that may be related to hormonal changes that come with aging. Concern over these changes may lead some men to seek information, but unfortunately, they may get their information from material designed to hype trendy products or promote sales. Information from these sources is often incorrect, leading to needless worry and unnecessary health problems.

The male sex hormone, testosterone, has been extensively studied for many decades. Its appropriate use and benefits to men with low hormonal levels are well documented. For this book, I have compiled scientific knowledge on the male sex hormones and related topics. It is written for men who have not had formal medical training but have a healthy curiosity about the workings of their own bodies. Much of the content for this book concerns the poorly understood but important subject of male sexuality.

This book is different because it's based on scientifically recognized information. As a physician, I view testosterone not as a miracle drug but as a new hope for men affected with low testosterone levels. Testosterone replacement treatment has the potential to help many men. It is possible that the use of testosterone by middle-aged and older men will eventually approach the widespread use of estrogen by menopausal women. I explore both the present and future states of testosterone research and its practical application. I have attempted to present a balanced review that includes the negative aspects of testosterone therapy as well as the positive.

I do advocate the use of testosterone when it is medically appropriate. My goal in this book is to provide a reliable, ethical, honest source of information about testosterone replacement therapy so that men, together with their physicians, can make informed choices.

CHAPTER ONE

Fountain of Youth

Masculinity, Testosterone, and the Aging Process

- Symptoms of Testosterone Deficiency
- Testosterone Deficiency and the Psychological Response to Aging
- Treating Testosterone Deficiency
- Benefits of Testosterone Replacement Treatment

W hat does "masculine" mean to men? Strong? Aggressive? Virile? Sexual? Well hung? Capable of rigid erections? Perhaps it means all these to some degree. There is no escaping the fact that the word *masculine* implies a combination of strength and sexuality to most men. A man's sense of his own masculinity is often the characteristic he values the most.

Young men tend to take their masculinity for granted, but as middle age approaches, they begin noticing a gradual decline in their physical vitality, strength, and sexual prowess. Men experience these age-related symptoms in the midst of society's pressures to maintain their youthfulness. Compounding this problem is the fact that men are naturally competitive. A man will compare himself to other men, wondering whether he's the only one experiencing these changes. He wants to know whether anything can be done to counteract the changes that come with aging, but he may be uncomfortable about seeking information.

Until now, little attention has been paid to the gradual changes that occur in men's bodies over time. While intense research into the role estrogen (the principal female sex hormone) plays in women has been going on since the 1920s, the role of testosterone in men has only recently received attention from researchers. Scientists have focused attention on estrogen deficiency because it has more obvious symptoms and is universal in older women, whereas testosterone deficiency has more subtle symptoms and affects fewer men. Declining estrogen levels (known as menopause) occur earlier and more dramatically in a woman's life, while the decline in testosterone in a man's life is slower and more subtle. But just as estrogen production falls off in women, so does testosterone production in men.

All men experience a gradual reduction of testosterone levels. Testosterone is the primary male sex hormone that influences physical vitality, development and maintenance of muscle mass, libido (sexual desire), erectile function, and sperm production. For men in their forties, the decrease is so small (about 1 percent per year) that it is almost imperceptible, even in laboratory tests. The decreased levels start to become noticeable in the fifth or sixth decade of life. The rate of decrease varies, and some men continue to make enough testosterone to support sexual function well into their nineties. Despite this, evidence suggests that as many as 60 percent of men over the age of fifty-five suffer some recognizable decrease in physical vitality, strength, and sexual prowess due to testosterone deficiency. This naturally occurring decline in testosterone levels can have a tremendous negative impact on the quality of men's lives as they approach middle age and beyond.

It is essential for men to gain an understanding of the advances in testosterone replacement treatment so that they may decide with their physician whether it will benefit them. Otherwise, a man may resign himself to an unfulfilling sexual life in his later years. The truth is that a healthy man can expect to be sexually active into the last decades of his life.

Symptoms of Testosterone Deficiency

Men who feel less "masculine" than they did in their younger years, who believe they are "losing it sexually," who have lost their zest for life, or who no longer have a feeling of well-being, should consider testosterone deficiency as a possible cause and seek medical attention for proper diagnosis and treatment.

Healthy testosterone levels are necessary for maintaining a man's libido (sexual desire). A man's baseline libido, established in his twenties, is usually the controlling factor of his lifetime sexual desire. For instance, a man who had intercourse frequently in his twenties will probably want it at only a slightly lesser frequency when he reaches middle age. When there is a testosterone deficiency, a man's libido can range from low to none compared to his baseline.

The most troublesome symptom associated with testosterone deficiency is the inability to develop and maintain penile erection for sexual intercourse. The various types of erection difficulties are extremely disturbing to men. They may complain, "It doesn't get as big as it used to," "It doesn't get as hard as it used to," "Halfway through I lose it—it goes soft," "It's too soft to get it in," or "I can't get hard no matter how much I try." Until recently, men rarely sought medical attention for erection difficulties, partly because of embarrassment and partly because of a lack of awareness about the variety of effective treatments that are now available. Another reason is that men may assume the problem is psychological in origin and not realize that their physician can help them.

Certain medical conditions other than testosterone deficiency can impact libido and erectile function. These include artery dysfunction, nerve dysfunction, and psychological difficulties. Declining sexual performance is also commonly related to other aging changes such as the onset of diabetes, the use of high blood pressure medication, or various treatments for prostate diseases. The symptoms of testosterone deficiency can mimic symptoms that are associated with other medical conditions such as thyroid disease, other hormone diseases, and chronic infections. Psychiatric conditions such as clinical depression, anxiety, and andropause ("male menopause") can also produce many of the same symptoms.

As one might expect, administration of testosterone for these other conditions is of no benefit, so a correct diagnosis of testosterone deficiency is essential. Blood tests for testosterone deficiency and pituitary gland disorders are readily available and reliable indicators of hormonal abnormalities. When a physician determines that the cause of erection difficulties is truly hormonal in nature, it will usually be due to a deficiency in testosterone and can be easily treated.

Testosterone Deficiency and the Psychological Response to Aging

Much confusion prevails about the differences between andropause (commonly known as "male menopause"), which is considered a psychological condition, and testosterone deficiency, which is considered a physical condition. These should be considered as separate conditions, although they do have some overlapping symptoms and occasionally can coexist. Because their treatments are different, it is very important that a man and his physician determine which of the two conditions is responsible for the symptoms. If the problem is both psychological and physical, then both will need treatment.

Diagnosis is complicated by the fact that andropause is often precipitated by physical changes. When a man becomes aware of age-related changes in his body such as reduced muscle performance and endurance, changes in his body contours, balding, and decreased vitality, he may slip into andropause. Such awareness of deteriorating physical health can be psychologically distressing. The physical changes can decrease a man's feeling of well-being. Therefore, anxiety, depression, and low self-esteem are common responses to testosterone deficiency.

The most common physical problem leading to andropause is impaired sexual performance, but the original cause of the problem may actually be a testosterone deficiency. Testosterone deficiency is easily diagnosed with a simple blood test; if it is ruled out, then psychological treatment directed at andropause is recommended.

Treating Testosterone Deficiency

Testosterone deficiency is totally reversible. The body's response to testosterone replacement treatment is very rapid, with men frequently noticing benefits within days.

The intensity of response to testosterone replacement treatment is in proportion to the severity of the hormone deficiency. If the blood level of testosterone is near zero, the effect of replacement treatment will be dramatic. If the blood concentration of testosterone is very low, the response will be pronounced. And if testosterone replacement is given for a low-normal blood level, a milder response will result.

Medical science is entering a new era in the understanding and treatment of testosterone deficiency. Drug companies and research labs are competing to bring out new developments in testosterone delivery systems. (Delivery systems refer to the way testosterone is actually introduced and absorbed into the body.) Now, more practical, convenient, effective, reliable, and safe delivery systems for testosterone are available. Testosterone is easily introduced into the body and has the same effect as that produced by the body itself. The action of the hormone is exactly the same, whether it comes from an external or internal source.

Most men are not yet aware of the benefits offered to them by scientific research and medical advances in testosterone replacement treatment. In their search for answers as to why they may be experiencing declines in vitality, strength, or sexual performance, men are exposed to information through the media that is misleading or inaccurate. Much of what men see and hear is designed to sell products that have been incompletely researched or verified. Some of the new trade books on "medical miracles" and life-enhancing and life-extending substances like DHEA (dehydroepiandrosterone) and hGH (human growth hormone) focus on the dramatic aspects of male hormones and are not based on solid scientific research. For men to make informed decisions about their bodies, they need accurate information, not anecdotal hype.

DHEA is one of the male sex hormones that has received attention in the media. It has less pronounced "masculinizing" effects than testosterone and aids in the synthesis of testosterone in the body. Recently, remarkable powers have been attributed to DHEA. The popularity and hype surrounding this hormone make it difficult to separate its real function from its placebo effect. The usefulness of DHEA in testosterone replacement treatment is unknown at this time. (A further discussion of DHEA appears in the Appendix.)

There are also synthetic male sex hormones (known as anabolic steroids) that produce effects very similar to those of testosterone. The goal in using anabolic steroids is to retain the muscle-building characteristics of testosterone without the other "masculinizing" and psychological side effects. Anabolic steroids are used principally by body builders. (Anabolic steroids are discussed in detail in Chapter 9.)

Benefits of
Testosterone Replacement Treatment

Is testosterone a "fountain of youth"? For many men, the answer is an emphatic yes. Testosterone replacement treatment can restore a man's testosterone level, and with it his sexuality and sense of masculinity, to that of a much younger man.

Testosterone replacement treatment can raise libido to the normal range. The increase in libido is immediately noticed and appreciated, and the entire spectrum of sexual response expands. A man becomes more sensuous as his visual, auditory, and tactile senses become more acute. With the correct dose of testosterone, a feeling of sexual need occurs more often and is more pervasive. His sex drive increases, thoughts of sex cross his mind more frequently, and the urge for sexual contact with his partner becomes more intense. His sexual partner may also experience benefits, such as feeling more desired and receiving more sexual attention and more frequent sexual contact.

For erection difficulties that are strictly due to testosterone deficiency, and when none of the other possible medical causes are present, testosterone replacement is usually effective in completely correcting the disorder and eliminating the symptoms. Of all the symptoms that are improved with hormonal replacement, the restoration of erectile function is the most satisfying and appreciated.

Testosterone replacement treatment can also increase physical vitality and muscle strength. Testosterone halts the shrinkage of muscles and eliminates muscle weakness. The overall mental attitude improves as the man becomes aware of the restoration of his normal physical and sexual functioning. The man may experience a renewed sense of general well-being and feel that the vigor and happiness of his younger years is returning. Adequate amounts of testosterone in the body can give a man a new lease on life.

CHAPTER TWO

The Virility Equation

How Testosterone Affects Men's Sex Lives

- Libido
- Testosterone and Libido
- Erection
- Orgasm
- Ejaculation

After the survival instinct, sexuality is the strongest of all human forces, with both its physical and mental aspects playing a dominant role in life from puberty on. Sex is not the special reserve of young men. A healthy man can realistically expect to be sexually active into the last decades of his life.

Male sexuality is directed by gonadal function and the male sex hormones, particularly testosterone. In puberty testosterone produces changes in the obvious masculine characteristics: a larger penis and scrotum, male-pattern pubic hair, a lower voice pitch, a male body configuration, greater bone and muscle structure, and an augmented libido.

Testosterone is also responsible for the mental and emotional changes of puberty. A boy perceives the increasing size of his genitalia and usually likes what he sees. He becomes aware of new penile sensations when manually stimulating his penis and enjoys masturbation. The libido-increasing effect of testosterone along with the hormone's structural effects initiates the adolescent boy into the wonderful world of sexuality. (See the Appendix for information on the influence of testosterone on growth and development.)

The male sex hormones play an extremely important role in all three of the basic male sexual functions: libido, erection, and orgasm. Testosterone directly impacts the intensity of a man's libido, his sensitivity and reaction to sexual stimulation of all kinds, the hardness and durability of his erection, and the frequency and strength of his orgasm. It also indirectly affects his sexuality by increasing his perceived sense of masculinity.

Beyond procreation and pleasure, sex offers additional benefits. Recent scientific research confirms that sex reduces stress and improves overall health. In addition, sexual pleasure can raise the pain threshold and even kill pain. People who have sex regularly are healthier physically and mentally than those who don't. And those who enjoy their sex lives also have been found to be altogether happier with their lives in general.

Libido

Horny, hot, excited, turned on, feeling sexy. These are all slang terms used to describe the libido that almost every man and woman recognizes. Libido is sexual desire—one's appetite for sexual gratification. Derived from the instinctive urge to procreate that is necessary for extending the survival of the species, it is the power that motivates the sex life.

Libido is the feeling of need for sexual satisfaction. Only the orgasm gratifies this sexual need. The sexual activities of hugging, kissing, stroking, and other stimulation (foreplay) without terminating in orgasm usually leave participants with a feeling of frustration and a greater need for sexual gratification.

The sexual appetite is very similar to the appetite for food. The longer the interval between meals, the hungrier one becomes. The intensity of the libido differs from one individual to another and at different times in a person's life. There is also variation in the type of appetite—what one craves. Some people are attracted to certain body builds or ethnic backgrounds or sexual orientation. Some need only a little sex to feel satisfied—a single orgasm—and others need considerably more—multiple orgasms. The amount of stimulation needed to achieve gratification also differs from person to person and situation to situation. Like food advertisements on television, visual and auditory exposure to erotic stimuli increases the appetite for sexual gratification in most people. An increase in testosterone levels in the body raises the libido at all ages in both men and women.

Libido is a function of a healthy mind and is controlled by the brain's limbic system, which is also associated with the control of emotions, eating, drinking, and sexual activity. Patients suffering with depression have a reduced libido and frequently have a total loss of their sexual drive. Sigmund Freud studied *libido* extensively as a part of sexuality and described it as a basic instinct. His use of the term carried much wider connotations than are ascribed to the word as it is generally used today. He believed that anxiety resulted from an accumulation of sexual tensions (or dammed-up libido) and neurosis from the holding back of libido. Carl Jung contended that libido was the unitary force of all psychic energy, not just the explicitly sexual.

There are no defined limits for what constitutes a normal libido. Some men normally have a low libido throughout their lives, desiring sex infrequently, whereas some men always need frequent sex to feel satisfied. A man's sex drive in later life, though somewhat reduced, is usually correlated to his libido in his younger years. For example, a young man who desires coitus or masturbation one or more times per day is likely to want sex twice a week in his sixties and seventies, but a man who wants sex twice a week in his thirties will probably be content with sexual gratification once a month in his senior years.

When a man is feeling libidinous, he is more likely to find what his senses tell him about a woman as sexy. Here is where testosterone enters the picture. During high libido, a man will find a greater percentage of women sexually attractive. When libido is low, all women look alike to him. Whether or not he takes action to gratify his needs with a particular woman depends on many things, such as his personality, circumstances, and past success or failure in his approach to women, but his lasciviousness is always a driving force.

Considerable differences exist between men and women as to their needs for sexual gratification. For both men and women a gradual waning of libido with aging is normal, but it never totally disappears. Some additional generalities can be made, keeping in mind that very wide variations within the normal ranges for both men and women are common.

Healthy women usually maintain a suitable libido level throughout their lifetime. The usual pattern is heightened sexuality in the late middle years and then a gradual decrease in the geriatric years. Women's libidos remain active even into their late eighties.

Regardless of libido level, women strongly prefer men to whom they are attracted for their sex partners. This attraction may be based on appearance, personality, respect, or a combination of these along with other characteristics. A woman desires sexual activity with someone who pleases her senses and feelings.

Men, on the other hand, can be satisfied sexually with women to whom they are not particularly attracted. Physical attraction often initiates the relationship, but it is not necessary for a man whose libido is active to experience gratification. So long as he doesn't find a woman's appearance repulsive, he is able to become sexually aroused and enjoy coitus with her. The physical gratification is equal to that experienced with a woman to whom he is attracted. There can be a great difference, however, in the emotional satisfaction he derives from sexual activity with a woman to whom he is attracted and one he is not.

A pretty woman with a nicely shaped body is attractive to almost every heterosexual man. But beyond this point there is very little agreement as to why a certain man finds a certain woman attractive. A large amount of psychological research is devoted to this subject. It is probably safe to say a man's response to different women depends on his lifetime experience with women. In other words, response is a learned process rather than a hardwired given. It's doubtful a man is born with a programmed sensitivity to specific types of women.

The learning process starts soon after birth and continues to death. Almost every experience with women, from casual acquaintanceship to intense love, influences a man's response both negatively and positively. Most of a man's concepts of sex begin during adolescence in the context of masturbation. His experiences and fantasies related to masturbation influence his lifetime sexual makeup.

The male libido is increased by other extrinsic factors in addition to testosterone levels. Abstinence, of course, is a significant factor, as is exposure to erotic stimuli. These points are well recognized and utilized by makers of movies and printed material. Both women and men are susceptible to visual and auditory sexual stimulation, but many people are offended by pornographic material, more often women than men. But women often respond to romantic stories and movies with increased libido as well. Body contact in dancing raises the libido, but this is considered more an arousal response than a libido response. In exposure to erotic stimuli and experience, determining where libido ends and arousal starts is difficult. When the libido is low, arousal will be delayed or absent.

Another fascinating psychological contrast between men and women is the difference in their feelings of, or desire for, closeness following coitus immediately after sex and during the days that follow. A woman is more likely than a man to seek continued physical and emotional closeness in this postcoital period.

This phenomenon is closely related to another difference between men and women. After coitus, a woman is inclined to feel more love and affection for her lover. Coitus can be the triggering factor where love starts, or, if love is already present, where love increases and becomes omnipresent. For a man, the long-term response depends on whether he loves the woman. If love is present, it will grow. If love is not present and he had intercourse purely for sexual gratification, he is likely to prefer to distance himself from the woman, both physically and emotionally, at least until the next time he is feeling libidinous.

Although adults usually recognize these disparities in female and male psychological characteristics, not all know how to deal with them and are ill prepared for these realities. Many need counseling to find relief from the miseries that these gender differences can create.

Testosterone and Libido

Testosterone production and the level of testosterone circulating in the blood have a powerful effect on the male libido. During the teen years, the level of testosterone rises steeply and parallels the libido. The beginning of decreased testosterone begins in a man's thirties (see Figure 2-1), but the decline is very gradual and minimal until the sixth decade in

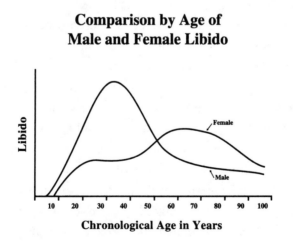

**Comparison by Age of
Male and Female Libido**

Figure 2-1. Comparison by age of male and female libido

the healthy male with normal testicular function. Reliable evidence indicates that libido also decreases when there is a significant drop in testosterone output from the testes. Men low in testosterone who receive testosterone replacement therapy (TRT) become sexually aroused with fewer and briefer extrinsic stimuli (see Chapter 5).

Scientists do not have a good explanation of how testosterone works on the mind to increase libido. They believe receptor sites in the brain respond to the testosterone molecules that are dispersed in the blood. The testosterone levels do not correspond exactly to the libido level. For example, the diurnal (daily) ups and downs of testosterone in the blood do not correlate with libidinal forces. Testosterone blood levels are the highest in the early morning hours, but libido varies throughout the day, though as men grow older this cyclic variation of testosterone decreases. As a man ages and the testosterone level falls, a gradual normal decrease in libido occurs, but aging and libido are not directly proportional.

The variation in levels of testosterone is one of the powerful determining factors in a man's libido. Whether a man is deficient or has a normal level of testosterone, extrinsically provided testosterone will heighten his libido. Scientific investigations certainly confirm testosterone given to men with gonad deficiency increases his libido. The hormone's effect on a man with normal gonad function is less clear as reported in current medical literature, but no doubt more about this response will be reported as testosterone comes into wider use.

The myth that highly libidinous men have a surge of hormone circulation is without foundation. No clinical evidence indicates that men with a high level of circulating testosterone have an abnormally high libido. Similarly, when adolescents show an interest in the opposite sex, it is not because they have unusually high hormonal levels. When men have a high blood level of testosterone from an inadvertently administered excess of testosterone, they show no evidence of an abnormal libido. Men who take very high doses of anabolic steroid compounds, which are pharmacologically related to testosterone, also do not demonstrate an unusual libido. They do show aggressiveness and tend to anger easily, but the abnormally high hormone level is not manifested in an increased libido.

Sexual addiction is a psychological concept, not a physical one. Medically speaking, there is no such thing as sexual addiction. Some healthy men and women with high libidos crave sexual activity more frequently than others, but their needs still fall within normal limits. Individuals whose sexual behavior falls outside these normal limits include those with psychiatric problems, such as nymphomania, and sex offenders. For these disturbed individuals, their sexual behavior is strongly influenced by factors other than libido.

Erection

The change of a flaccid penis to an erect and ready organ is one of the most complex physiological functions of the human body. It requires an interplay among the psyche, the nervous system, arteries, veins, muscles, and hormones. If any one element of this system fails, erection does not occur or is lost during sexual intercourse.

It is possible to achieve an erection solely by physical stimulation of the penis without the accompaniment of erotic thoughts. The friction from tight clothing or bedding while asleep is enough to cause an erection. But in the absence of direct physical stimuli, the mind triggers the beginning of an erection. The mental event can be at either the conscious or subconscious level. When it occurs at the conscious level, it is a response to a sensory stimulus. The stimulus may be visual, auditory, tactile (touch), or any combination of these. For some, the sense of smell can contribute to the triggering. The stimulus creates a nerve impulse sent by the brain, down the spinal cord, and out to the various blood vessels and tissues involved in erection.

An erection begins when the nerve impulses, from the brain to the walls of the arteries entering the penis, alter the flow of blood to the organ. At the beginning of an erection, the blood in the arteries flows at a rate exceeding 100 milliliters (more than three ounces) per minute. The extra flow fills special blood compartments called *sinusoids*. The filled pouches press on the soft walls of the return veins, closing them off so the blood cannot escape.

The rising of a penis is due to the distention of the walls within the penis and can be compared with what happens to an empty balloon when blown up. Where the penis joins the pelvic bone, a short but strong fibrous structure called the *suspensory ligament* attaches that part of the penis to the bone. This ligament determines the "angle of the dangle" and points the penis upward during erection. As men age, the suspensory ligament elongates and loses some of its tensile strength.

The degree of hardness of erection needed for insertion (penetration or intromission) depends on the angle of approach, the size of the erect penis, whether there is hand assistance by the man or his partner, the degree of vaginal lubrication, and the size of the woman's *introitus* (entrance). The size of a woman's introitus increases with sexual excitement when the muscles of the entrance become more relaxed. The introitus is smaller in women who have not borne children or who have had their deliveries by cesarean section. This small size is accentuated after menopause. Even a soft penis, if large enough, can be inserted with cooperation and effort. Referred to as "stuffing," this act accomplishes very little for either the man or his partner, although occasionally the penis will become erect.

During an erection, the skin covering the penis is soft and pliable, but the underlying structures become almost as hard as a bone. In rare instances, a semierect penis is sufficient for an orgasm, but almost always an erect penis is necessary for a man to experience an orgasm. The erect penis during coitus senses the massaging effect on the *glans* (the cap-shaped extension at the end of the penis) and transmits appropriate nerve impulses to nerves and tissues involved in orgasm (ejaculation). The flaccid penis has much less sensitivity.

If a man's mind becomes distracted by something threatening, such as physical danger or a physical threat, his erect penis immediately becomes flaccid. Any interruption of sexual activity—for instance, by an intruder—results in an almost immediate end to an erection. The route of impulses is the same as that which begins the erection. The mind sends a message to the spinal cord and on to the pelvis and penis to remove the obstruction of blood flow from the penis. The blood that engorged the penis is immediately dumped back into the bloodstream.

Erection difficulties are common among men of all ages. Even the teenager whose mind is diverted loses his erection, but frequent loss of erection without cause is not prevalent. The most frequent cause of erection difficulties in healthy men over fifty is a mental block, and the most common form of mental block is fear of failure. The mind is focused on the hardness of the penis instead of love, affection, sex, and the good feeling. Poor health can also contribute to erection loss, as can medications that block the erection reflex. For good erection function, men, especially older men, must feel good about themselves. It helps greatly if they feel strong and robust and are satisfied with their bodies (in other words, if they feel masculine.

Testosterone and Erection

Physicians and researchers generally agree that testosterone improves a man's outlook on his life, increases his well-being. This translates into a feeling of strength and masculinity. A positive attitude about one's self, plus the driving force of high libido, results in greater erectile powers. In simple terms, testosterone sets the mental scene for better erectile function. Most physicians treating impotence order testosterone blood tests early in the evaluation process because they know improving erection powers is difficult in the presence of low testosterone levels.

Medical researchers have yet to fully explain testosterone's role in the process of penile erection. It is possible that the presence of adequate amounts of the hormone are needed for more than one stage of the erectile function. It may be that the thinking part of the mind, when there is a feeling of well-being, gives favorable signals to the hypothalamus. Scientific investigation will hopefully be able to answer these and other questions in the future.

Testosterone is helpful in treating erection difficulties at any age, especially if the hormone levels are low. Erection may occur in the absence of testosterone, but the frequency is less and usually less firmness results. Prepubescent boys, though producing very little testosterone, have frequent erections;

even newborn babies have them. Castrated animals, such as stallions, continue to have sizable erections.

Obviously, a man who seeks to improve erection function would do well to develop good health habits such as eating a balanced diet, avoiding excesses of alcohol, not using tobacco, getting regular aerobic exercise, and possibly starting a weight training program. Positive mental practices are also beneficial. These include reducing stressors and following a lifestyle that promotes happiness, contentment, and peace of mind.

Some men use extrinsic means to bolster their sense of machismo (masculinity), which results in better sexual performance. Classical examples are purchasing a sports car or having a relationship with a younger partner. This syndrome, called *andropause,* is discussed in Chapter 7. Unfortunately, these are temporary, Band-Aid fixes. The improvement in erection function is usually short-lived and can sometimes lead to disaster.

Orgasm

An orgasm is an intense, subjective, emotional event that typically corresponds to a man's ejaculation. Orgasm is a mentally perceived experience, whereas ejaculation is a physical function. But they are intimately related, as every man knows.

The word *orgasm* is often used interchangeably with *ejaculation,* but this usage is a mistake because one can occur without the other. An example is the normal orgasm after prostate surgery during which there is no ejaculation. Ejaculation refers to the sudden act of expulsion of the semen. Orgasm is the apex and culmination of sexual excitement. The word *climax* refers to orgasm but has been used less commonly in recent years. Whereas libido is a mental function and erection is a physical function, orgasm is a combination of mental and physical functions.

The psychological elements of orgasm are not well understood but are an important part of orgasm. Orgasm requires intense, very focused mental concentration. The mind becomes closed to extrinsic thoughts and must be intensely directed toward sex. As thoughts becomes more and more concentrated on sexual matters, the closer a person comes to the time of orgasm. Any interruption of this emotional crescendo can prevent orgasm. The more intent a person's mind is on erotic thoughts, the sooner and stronger is the orgasm.

Any disruption of the mental process can slow the arrival of the orgasm or totally prevent it. Disruptions can be intrinsic, such as pain, or extrinsic, such as an unexpected sound. The disruption concept has been used to slow down premature ejaculation. This technique involves the man or his partner pinching a certain part of the penis just as the orgasm is about to begin. Unfortunately, it's not very effective in most cases so is not used much.

Erotic thoughts encourage "good" orgasms. These thoughts may be produced by visual, auditory, or tactile stimuli. For example, sexual encouragement by way of caresses or words ("dirty talk") can amplify an orgasm. The stimulus can also take the form of fantasy. Some women learn to use their internal pelvis muscle to produce an improved orgasmic response with a massaging effect. Some partners use anal stimulation to create a higher level of excitement and stronger orgasms.

How "good" an orgasm is depends on one or more of these features: intensity of muscle contractions in the pelvic, trunk, and extremity muscles; duration of the orgasm; number of spasms experienced during orgasm; erotic concentration; responsiveness of the partner; and the amount of relaxation of the body muscles after coitus. The first three factors are objective and measurable; the last three are subjective. Overall, a subjective evaluation determines the quality of an orgasm.

The length of time between stimulation and orgasm (ejaculation) varies greatly from one man to another and for an individual at different times, and it is affected by several factors, both physical and psychological. In general, the younger one is, the briefer the interval. In the adolescent this time period may be as short as a few seconds, but for a man in his eighties it may be as long as thirty to forty minutes. The strength and vigor of young men shorten the interval, while the reduced strength and endurance of older or chronically ill men lengthen it. The aging process extends this period of time by reducing the sensory nerve function in the penis. This condition is most commonly due to impaired circulation to the nerve tissue. Prevention is the best way to avert the problem by avoiding things that damage the arteries such as tobacco, obesity, high blood pressure, and untreated diabetes.

The force of the libido also affects the duration of the interval between stimulation and orgasm. Young men can hardly wait to have an orgasm because of the subconscious driving force of an active libido. In older men who are low in testosterone, the duration may be longer than desired. Testosterone replacement therapy can be useful in this case. The hormone shortens the interval by increasing libido and heightening vigor.

Some older men normally fail to have an orgasm, sometimes even after having a full erection. There is less compulsion to have an orgasm when there is less tension in the mind and muscle built up during the excitement stage of coitus.

Coitus without orgasm still can be satisfying to an older, loving man, especially if his partner has an orgasm.

Women's Orgasm and Sexuality

A woman can also experience satisfaction after coitus even without orgasm if she feels love and affection and knows she has provided pleasure for her lover.

In some cases, when stimulation or thrusting is stopped before a woman reaches orgasm, she may experience feelings of anxiety that extend for twenty-four hours or more. This feeling coincides with pelvic congestion (distention of the large veins in the pelvis) in a woman's body during sexual excitement. At orgasm the blood is released back into the bloodstream, corresponding to the flow of blood from the male penis after orgasm. A woman can have an unpleasant sensation of fullness or heaviness in her pelvis after anorgasmic sexual activity. The frustration and pelvic congestion do not occur if she has been adequately stimulated.

Orgasm experiences and patterns are just as variable in women as in men. In general, a woman who can achieve orgasm in early adulthood will continue to have numerous and gratifying orgasms in her later years provided she is physically and psychologically healthy. Unfortunately, many older women have been led to believe sex is not part of life for the aged and so suppress their thoughts of sex. But a healthy woman may be sexually active throughout life, although this activity varies greatly. Past patterns of sexuality influence the sexuality patterns in later life. The woman who enjoys or needs sexual gratification frequently in early years of adulthood will more likely remain sexually active in her geriatric years.

How active a female is depends on a number of factors. A woman needs a healthy, sexually attractive sex partner to maintain her interest in sex. Her natural instinct to remain sexually active can readily be suppressed if her partner is impotent or shows little interest in coitus. In their advanced years many men are physically incapable of penetration because of chronic disease or medications. Interestingly, if a woman who has been indifferent to sex loses her sexually inactive husband through death or divorce, she may very soon become interested in sex and sexually active with a new partner.

A woman's own health is also a strong contributing factor. Chronic illness and debility reduce interest in sex. Many older women are physically unable to participate in coitus because of shrinkage of the vagina, which can be prevented with estrogen replacement. With replacement the vagina remains physically receptive. The good mental attitude produced by estrogen replacement therapy is also conducive to greater interest in sexual activity.

Testosterone and Orgasm

Testosterone plays an important role in orgasms. In adequate levels it promotes the health and responsiveness of the body's organs and tissues involved in ejaculation. Testosterone is necessary to the development of these structures but is not entirely necessary to maintain their function.

Testosterone establishes a feeling of well-being and happiness. A dysphoric person is pessimistic about his day-to-day performance, whether it be in his occupation or his personal life. With testosterone boosting his spirits, his mind is more capable of facilitating a satisfactory orgasm. Not only will the man himself be aware of better orgasms, but his sexual partner will appreciate the improvement also. Each sexual partner enjoys participating in a gratifying sexual experience for the other. Because of increased libido caused by testosterone, a man feels a greater need for the pleasure and gratification of orgasm. As libido increases, the compulsion for orgasm increases. Testosterone also strengthens a man's muscles and improves his self-esteem, which in turn makes him a more vigorous lover. This wonderful mental stimulus improves his orgasmic power. His thoughts are more in tune with the driving force leading to a successful orgasm.

Ejaculation

Emission and ejaculation are responses to sympathetic nerve actions but are also influenced by androgen levels. The brain centers for emission or ejaculation are controlled by dopamine and serotonin. These are chemicals made by the body that act as neurotransmitters by carrying messages through nerve tissues. Dopamine, by way of nerve channels, is conducive to the brain activity for orgasm. Serotonin, on the other hand, acts via nerve channels that slow or obstruct nerve control of orgasm.

After orgasm, when the penis becomes flaccid, there is a time interval before a new erection can occur. This time interval is called the *resolution phase* but more correctly the *refractory period*. It is longer for men than women. The duration of this time period varies greatly from one individual to another and from one orgasm to another, depending on the intensity of the orgasm. *Detumescence* (softening) is slower when the penis is allowed to stay in the vagina than if immediately withdrawn after ejaculation. It may not completely detumesce if left in the vagina for many minutes.

Several factors determine the duration of the resolution phase—chiefly, age, general health, libido, the day-to-day fluctuations in lifestyle, and feeling of well-being. The inability to get another erection immediately after orgasm is also partly due to simple mental and physical fatigue of the big, complex muscles involved during the excitement phase of orgasm.

Young men are capable of twenty to thirty orgasms in a twenty-four hour period, but most of them are satisfied with five to ten per day. At the other end of the spectrum, men in their eighties might have only one orgasm a month. There is a difference between what an individual is capable of and what he prefers, and there is a wide variation in both normal limits and preferences. The limiting factor is the refractory time in the resolution phase.

The highest concentration of sperm is in the first ejaculate after an abstinence of twenty-four to seventy-two hours. Because the organs produce their secretions fairly steadily, the volume of the ejaculated semen decreases as the ejaculations come closer together. Organs of secretion are the testes, seminal vesicles, prostate, and other less active tissues. When no ejaculation occurs for a day, the next masturbation or coitus will produce two to five milliliters of ejaculate, which will be expelled with significant force, shooting twelve to twenty-four inches. With each succeeding ejaculation, both the amount and the force decrease. By the fourth or fifth ejaculation, the volume is reduced to two or three drops that slowly ooze from the urethra. In a man's more advanced years, both the volume and the force are less, but fortunately this change does not detract significantly from the pleasure of orgasm.

CHAPTER THREE

Never Too Old

The Effects of Aging on Male Hormone Production

- **Aging Effects on Testosterone**
- **A Medical View**
- **Antiaging Remedies**

O urs is a culture obsessed with youth. Ageism is on the increase, with older people regarded in many ways as second-class citizens. Like death and taxes, however, aging is a fact of life.

Aging means different things to different people. Many think of it as the deteriorating changes in appearance and bodily functions that occur in later life. In medical terms, it refers to the entire process of change from time of conception to time of death. At some stages in life, aging is a desirable change. Teenagers want to age rapidly so they can have the rights of an adult, such as dating and driving a car.

But at the other end of the life span, aging is not considered in our culture as a desirable change. No matter how healthy the lifestyle, bodies and minds eventually record the passing of time. Even professional athletes must accept the aging process and retire when the blood supply to the nervous system diminishes, slowing their reflex time and reducing the strength in their muscles. In some parts of the body, the aging process begins as early as twenty, but most men start noticing the cumulative changes sometime in their forties.

The physiological changes in aging men are more subtle than those in women. As men grow older, their sexual function starts to decline. Their equipment still operates, but it is less vigorous than when they were younger. The bones lose density, muscles begin to atrophy, and pockets of fat collect around the middle of the torso.

Aging Effects on Testosterone

Younger men take their masculinity and virility for granted, but as men reach midlife and start noticing their strength decreasing and their sexual prowess waning, they want to know whether anything can be done to slow or counteract the physical decline that accompanies aging.

Men do not experience the abrupt physical and sexual changes women undergo in menopause, so little attention has been paid to the more gradual changes in the masculine body. But just as estrogen production falls off in women, so does testosterone production in men, but not as precipitously (see Figure 3-1). The abrupt and radical decrease in women's hor-

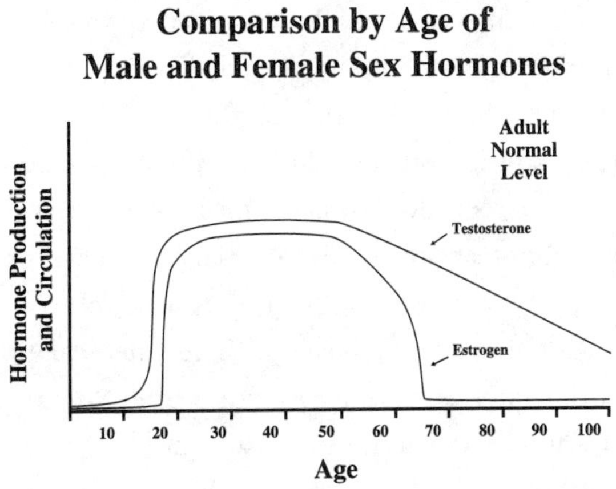

Comparison by Age of
Male and Female Sex Hormones

Figure 3-1. Comparison by age of male and female hormone levels

mones around age fifty is responsible for menopause. Male sex hormones decrease very gradually over decades, so the changes men experience as a result tend to be less dramatic.

Every sixteen seconds a man in the United States turns fifty, which means that in the next decade, nineteen million men will be that age. Currently, twenty-five million men suffer some degree of impotence. By age seventy, 25 percent of all men are impotent. Men start to run low on some hormones after forty, and their testosterone declines steadily over the next thirty years. The decrease in testosterone leads to a reduction in muscle, bone mass, and height as well as some sexual dysfunction for the majority.

Between the ages of forty and seventy, an average man may lose anywhere from twelve to twenty pounds of muscle and two inches in height. His sperm production declines, and his testicles become smaller. By age sixty, testosterone levels have dropped to the low end of normal. The sexual and reproductive systems still work, but the pituitary gland transmits weaker orders to the testicles, where fewer cells are available to respond. A 15 percent loss of bone mass also occurs. It is well documented that testosterone is necessary to retard the universal condition of osteoporosis, but the exact level to do so has not been adequately established. The medical literature abounds with evidence showing fractures are most common in older men who are deficient in testosterone.

Studies show that the bioavailable (active) testosterone falls from 40 to 65 percent in normal men as they age, although not all research confirms this result. The greatest output of testosterone occurs for most men around age thirty. From then on there is an extremely gradual drop in testosterone levels, with the rate of decline accelerating slightly at about age fifty. Then the rate of decrease is fairly steady at about 1 percent a year for the rest of the lives of healthy, normal men, declining about 30 to 40 percent by age seventy. But there is considerable variation in the pattern, probably related to a man's general health status and lifestyle.

The cause of decreased testosterone levels in aging men is thought to be mainly due to testicular failure associated with atherosclerosis. (See the Appendix for a discussion of atherosclerosis.) Another cause suggested by a recent study is the high prevalence (48 percent) in men over the age of fifty of secondary hypogonadism, which causes a low bioavailability of testosterone. *Secondary hypogonadism* means some cause outside the testicles themselves is present, such as chronic or acute illness, injury to scrotal contents, or medications with side effects on the testes.

The most common cause of the gradual reduction in testosterone levels, as with many age-related changes, is the reduced blood flow through the arteries, although there are a number of other, more subtle reasons. When the blood flow through the testes starts diminishing, the activity of the two kinds of cells in the testes also lessens. The Sertoli cells produce fewer and fewer spermatozoa, and the Leydig cells produce less and less testosterone. As the Leydig cells decrease in number, the output of testosterone decreases. With increasing age, the number of Leydig cells declines and the response in receptor cells diminishes, causing an increase in hormones produced by the pituitary gland—follicle stimulating hormone (FSH) and luteinizing hormone (LH). There is a complex explanation for this involving other hormones. As men age, sex hormone binding globulin (SHBG) increases, which renders testosterone less active.

As the blood flow decreases, a man loses his fertility and is decreasingly likely to father a baby. Thirty million sperm are produced daily from puberty to death. The number of sperm produced does not significantly drop with aging, but sperm motility, one of the indices determining reproduction level, decreases. The number of deformed sperm also rises as men age.

The effects of decreasing testosterone levels on sexual function are often overstated. Declining sexual activity is more commonly related to other aging changes such as the onset of diabetes, the use of high blood pressure medication, and treatments for prostate diseases. In men under age forty-five, the incidence of impotency is 5 percent but rises to 50 percent in men over seventy-five; however, 90 percent of these have other medical conditions or take medication that is responsible for the impotency.

A Medical View

Testosterone deficiency is not considered a state of wellness. Dorland's medical dictionary defines *disease* as "any deviation from or interruption of the normal structure or function of any part, organ or system of the body." It does not qualify as to age. *Illness* is defined as "a condition marked by pronounced deviation from the normal healthy state"—again, no mention of age. The disadvantages of doing nothing about it are similar to the disadvantages of not using estrogen replacement. Bones deteriorate; abnormalities of the genitalia and their function develop; the feeling of well-being is lost.

Testosterone deficiency is a natural transition, but it does not mean that men should suffer the consequences. Consider that physicians treat other aging conditions without clear-cut evidence of deficiencies or abnormalities. A person who has joint discomfort, for example, is often treated with anti-inflammatory medication on suspicion of early arthritis even though X-rays and blood tests are normal. Many physicians prescribe estrogen for a woman having mild menopausal symptoms (hot flashes, dry vagina) even though estrogen deficiency is not apparent in the physical examination.

Administering testosterone to aging men is called *testosterone replacement therapy* (TRT). It is one remedy that physicians recognize as both useful and valuable, though some unethical providers still promote testosterone as a miracle drug and make promises of benefits beyond what has been proven.

All men have a natural reduction in testosterone production, but the rate of fall is highly variable. Reasons for the decrease are both intrinsic (artery disease, diabetes, other gland dysfunction) and extrinsic (infections, injury, surgery).

Most men accept the changes that come with age and falling testosterone levels. They expect to become weaker and for their sexuality to diminish somewhat with age. They make up the 80 to 95 percent of men who either don't need or don't want testosterone replacement therapy. But those who find a widening gap between their own and their partner's sexuality, and those who miss their sense of well-being, might benefit from TRT. (See Chapter 5 for a discussion of TRT.)

Antiaging Remedies

The will to survive is the strongest of all human forces, and the fight to retard aging is part of that force. Even before Ponce de Leon set sail for Bimini to find the fountain of youth, people had been longing and searching for a means of stopping or retarding the aging process. Today more opportunities and more interactions exist for people who are healthy and active, and consequently the longing has greatly intensified the searching. Organizations are popping up, like the Longevity Institute and the American Academy of Antiaging Medicine, that focus on finding or producing youthening substances. The search for eternal youth has generated a multibillion-dollar industry as profiteers work feverishly to manufacture and sell those remedies. While some are widely accepted and prescribed by professionals, other products and services promoted as antiaging remedies are of no value and can even be harmful.

Essentially two categories of antiaging drugs are currently available. The first and larger category is composed of drugs that affect specific organs or tissues. Some of these organ-specific drugs reverse the aging changes, such as Rogaine,

Mevacor, and Proscar. Others reduce or eliminate aging symptoms but do not reverse or retard the actual process of aging, such as estrogen, testosterone, and Retin-A.

Organ-specific drugs that reverse aging changes include the following:

Rogaine. This is a popular hair preparation that rejuvenates the hair follicles and retards hair loss due to aging. It does not, however, restore luxuriant growth.

Some cholesterol-lowering drugs. These drugs reverse the narrowing of the coronary arteries and the symptoms that result from reduced blood flow. Mevacor (Lovastatin), Niacin, Lopid (Gemfibrozil), Zocor (Simvastin), Pravachol (pravastatin), Lipitor (Atorvastatin), and Lescol (Fluvastatin) are products that may reverse the cholesterol accumulation in the coronary artery walls, allowing greater blood flow and possibly decreasing angina (chest pain) and the likelihood of a myocardial infarction (heart attack).

Proscar (Finateride). This medication stops or retards benign prostate enlargement. It helps decrease the related urinary bladder symptoms almost all men experience with aging. Proscar actually stops this aging process, going beyond just stopping the symptoms.

Organ-specific drugs that reduce or eliminate aging symptoms but don't reverse or retard the actual process of aging include these:

Topical skin preparations. Examples of these products include Effudex (Flurouracil) and Retin-A (Tretinoin), which work to eliminate recent changes such as wrinkling and discoloration. These products produce a younger appearance although the skin continues to age.

Estrogen for women. The aging of a woman's ovaries cannot be prevented or retarded, but the universally recognized symptoms of estrogen deficiency can be effectively eliminated by estrogen replacement.

Testosterone for men. Testicular failure is a gradual but real aging change in almost all men. Nothing will reverse or retard the reduction of testosterone from the testes, but effective replacement therapy for the symptoms is available.

The second and smaller category of antiaging drugs target the entire body rather than a specific organ. This group of drugs has been commanding a lot of media attention because of its appeal to consumers. In many cases, the results promised by advertising campaigns are not based on any sort of thorough scientific studies. Authors, entrepreneurs, and drug companies, looking for notoriety or profit, often make claims for drugs that cannot be substantiated, and, in some cases, they are not disclosing potentially harmful side effects. Unethical producers and promoters of drugs take just a smidgen of the research information and use it to sell their products. This category includes antioxidants and DHEA.

Antioxidants and Aging

Considerable interest and research over the past few years has focused on the activity of *free radicals*. Generally speaking, free radicals are oxygen atoms that have a deficiency of one electron. Because of the one-electron deficiency, a free radical is more likely to attach itself or combine with other chemicals.

This oxygen bonding constitutes one type of oxidation. In the body, oxidation accelerates aging in various tissues—or so the theory goes. Some early studies suggest that slowing oxidation by reducing the number of free radicals might reduce the beginning and/or progression of various diseases such as cancer. The most widely recognized antioxidants are beta carotene (one form of vitamin A), vitamins C and E, and the minerals zinc and selenium.

Some valid research suggests that the antioxidants do retard a few aging symptoms, but very little information is available on their ability to retard the aging of the testes. Moreover, a few recent studies have introduced some skepticism into the favorable surge for antioxidants. One research team found that vitamin E had no effect whatever on the occurrence of lung cancer. Another reported an 8 percent higher mortality rate, mostly from lung cancer and coronary heart disease, in those taking beta carotene. An unusually high number of hemorrhagic strokes among vitamin E users has also been noted. It is possible that vitamin E interferes with normal blood clotting. Many research projects on antioxidants are in progress, but they are far from completion.

Antioxidants include some phytochemicals, most of which have been available over the counter for many years. The word *phytochemical* designates newly discovered, or expected-to-be-discovered, substances in foods that benefit the body. The term usually refers to minute amounts of chemicals found in fruits and vegetables that have not yet achieved the status of vitamins. The suspected presence of such chemicals has led to the concept that eating fruits and vegetables is better than taking vitamins in pill form. For the most part, phytochemicals are safe even when taken in large doses. They have a slow onset of action in the body so the benefits are not immediately apparent. The physical changes occur so gradually that the user is seldom aware of the effects.

Claims have also been made for superhormones, human growth hormone, and melatonin, but there's insufficient research on which to base conclusions. The interest in these substances was originally based on ethical laboratory studies, but the resulting data have been improperly expanded or applied.

DHEA and Aging

A plethora of articles and books extol the antiaging benefits of taking supplemental DHEA (dihydroepiandrosterone), a naturally occurring male hormone. Early research with animals found an association between DHEA and a healthier, longer life and an inhibition in the development of atherosclerosis. Studies on humans are currently being conducted in several medical centers. Early results seem to indicate that DHEA encourages stronger and larger muscles, especially in the upper body, along with a decrease in fat deposits. The most dramatic effect reported is in users' moods. The improved mood translates in higher energy levels and improved memory and mental agility. The increased libido reported by DHEA users is probably related to better mood but may also be due to a more direct effect.

There are obvious similarities between the effects claimed for DHEA and those of testosterone. Both increase muscle size and strength, and both intensify the libido and provide a feeling of well-being. The degree of benefits observed seems to be dose related. Because DHEA and testosterone are chemically similar (see the Appendix), it is not surprising that they have similar effects on the body. But the similarities include the side effects as well as the benefits.

The potential side effects from DHEA are worrisome. DHEA is usually taken orally. Soon after it is swallowed, it enters the liver and may have some adverse effects on that organ, just as orally taken testosterone does in some men. Liver damage is also a recognized side effect of orally taken anabolic steroids, which are also chemically and pharmacologically related to testosterone and DHEA. Because DHEA is an androgen, it is possible that, like testosterone, it may also stimulate growth in prostate cancers.

The androgenic side effects of DHEA are particularly hazardous for women and may include acne, hair loss, hirsutism (excessive and abnormal hair growth), and deepening of the voice. The latter two effects appear to be irreversible.

At this time, the FDA has not approved DHEA for human use. But the hormone is available over the counter when labeled as a dietary supplement. Until more research results are published, it is doubtful that many physicians will prescribe DHEA for their patients. In the meantime, the *Medical Letter on Drugs and Therapeutics* (vol. 38, Oct. 11, 1996) recently concluded, "There is no convincing evidence that DHEA has any beneficial effects on aging or on any disease. Patients would be well advised not to take it." (See the Appendix for a further discussion of DHEA.)

CHAPTER FOUR

Diminishing Supplies

Causes and Effects of Testosterone Deficiency

- **Causes of Testosterone Deficiency**
- **Testosterone Deficiency and Aging**
- **Testosterone Deficiency and Sexuality**
- **Testosterone Deficiency and Osteoporosis**
- **Testosterone Deficiency and Depression**
- **Testosterone Deficiency and Changes in Memory and Cognition**

Normal testosterone levels in men vary by as much as 20 to 50 percent on a daily basis. The highest levels occur between 6 and 9 A.M., followed by a progressive decline over the duration of the day. Some men's testosterone switches to an afternoon peak in the late fall and early winter. And during puberty, young men often have rises in their testosterone

Normal Range of Testosterone Levels by Age (in nanograms per deciliter of blood)	
<2 weeks	2–350 ng/dl
<1 year	2–7 ng/dl
1–5 years	2–25 ng/dl
6–9 years	3–30 ng/dl
10–11 years	5–50 ng/dl
12–14 years	10–572 ng/dl
15–17 years	220–800 ng/dl
>17 years	280–1,100 ng/dl

levels during sleep. Testosterone levels in men over sixty-five appear to be much more stable and less affected by daily fluctuations.

One postulation as to why testosterone levels in newborns is so high and then slacks off is that there is an abrupt and extreme drop in the hormones circulating from the mother's blood, so there is a parallel drop in the baby's hormones. The extremely high female hormone levels suppress the pituitary hormones that hold gonad activity in check. When the female hormones drop in the newborn, the pituitary senses this, and an outpouring of their stimulating secretion results, demanding a much greater output of testosterone.

By far the most common symptom of falling testosterone levels, and the one that most often motivates a visit to a doctor, is the alteration in a man's sexual function. The change might be as insignificant as a reduction in sexual appetite or as serious as an inability to maintain an erection or achieve orgasm. But testosterone deficiency has other serious, if less dramatic symptoms. The symptoms of insufficient testosterone are consistent regardless of the cause of the deficiency.

Causes of Testosterone Deficiency

The vast majority of cases of testosterone deficiency can be attributed to normal aging changes in the circulation to the gonads (see Chapter 3). As the arteries constrict with age, the blood supply to the testosterone-producing Leydig cells in the gonads diminishes, and less testosterone is produced. For most men, this is not a debilitating change; but in others, the amount of circulating testosterone drops below an acceptable level, producing symptoms that are serious enough to require medical intervention.

Contrary to popular opinion, vasectomies and cancer of the prostate do not suppress testosterone production. Some other, mostly rare, conditions can impair or completely suppress testosterone production, yielding the same symptoms as an age-related reduction in testosterone (see the Appendix).

Injury to the testes is uncommon because they are so well protected, but it is possible to sustain an injury such as torsion (twisting of the chord to the testes) that would affect testosterone production if left untreated. It is also possible to sustain an injury to the testicle blood supply. Surgical procedures such as hernia repairs rarely impair the blood supply to the testes, but inadvertent disruption can occur even when surgery is performed by the best of surgeons under the best of conditions.

Castration, the complete removal or closure of the testes, lowers testosterone levels. It is performed occasionally for the treatment of certain advanced cancers such as prostate cancer. Castration reduces the body's testosterone abruptly. It does not totally prevent the body's testosterone production capacity but is definitely sufficient to slow down the progression of prostate cancer. (See the Appendix for a further discussion of castration.)

Testosterone Deficiency and Aging

In older men, there is only a subtle difference between the effects of reduced testosterone levels due to normal aging changes and the symptoms of abnormal testosterone deficiency. In younger men, the difference is quite pronounced. Men whose bodies are deficient in testosterone have both physical and mental indications. The psychological symptoms are, at least partially, the result of a man's reactions to the physical disturbances.

Men who have lost their zest for life and experience a decrease in their feeling of well-being, who have become less productive, feel less masculine, notice muscle strength waning, become aware of angst or depression, note a lower self-esteem, or believe they're "losing it" sexually, would be wise to consider testosterone deficiency as an explanation for these developments. (See Chapter 5 for a discussion of testosterone replacement therapy.)

Most men like to have large or at least average-sized muscles. Many men take great joy in their large pectorals and quadriceps. They relate muscle configuration to masculinity. The bigger the muscles, the more masculine they feel. A few men probably engage in muscle building to improve their health, but the rest are striving for an appearance of strength and masculinity. The desire for strong, large muscles has created an enormous muscle-enhancing industry in the United States.

Testosterone deficiency causes muscle weakness and shrinkage. When a man, who all of his life has taken pride in a strong, well-shaped body, develops testosterone deficiency with the associated muscle deterioration, he naturally becomes unhappy about it. With the shrinkage of muscles, a man feels less attractive to others and less masculine. If this reduced sense of masculinity is accompanied by a reduction of sexuality, the results are predictable—the man's self-image, both physical and mental, deteriorates.

Testosterone deficiency also produces a decrease in vigor and aggressiveness. Vigor reflects the intensity of body and mental force. In the medical literature on testosterone, the words *vigor* and *aggressiveness* are usually paired. The term *aggressiveness,* when describing the effects of testosterone, means a driving, forceful energy or initiative. Throughout their productive years, men enjoy and benefit by feeling and acting vigorous. It gives them an advantage in the workplace and adds pleasure to their work efforts. Success in life is often a result of aggressive behavior; a competitive nature improves a man's chance of achieving his goals. When a man who has enjoyed vigor and good mental and physical health becomes testosterone deficient, these qualities begin to dwindle. The change is disturbing and the loss becomes devastatingly more apparent.

Hot flashes due to falling testosterone levels with age are extremely rare and, when they do occur, are infrequent and mild in severity. It is speculated that men don't experience hot flashes because of the very slow rate of fall in testosterone as compared with the rate of fall of estrogen in women. Men are more likely to have hot flashes when there is an abrupt, marked fall, as in those who are castrated for the treatment of advanced prostate cancer. Men can feel excessive warmth from systemic conditions such as an overly active thyroid gland (hyperthyroidism) or from psychological disturbances. However, if a man reports hot flashes, he should be tested for possible testosterone deficiency as well as other causes.

Testosterone Deficiency and Sexuality

Testosterone deficiency unquestionably decreases men's sexuality. Sexuality includes more than the ability to have sexual intercourse. It also entails the expression of sexual receptivity or interest such as choice of words and manner of speaking, appearance, clothing, posture, and body language. When a man arrives at the doctor's office and complains of sex problems, although he may be referring to a particular relationship, most often he is referring to a decreased libido, less interest in sex, erection failure, or unsatisfactory orgasms. Regardless of his description of sexual impairment, he is an unhappy man. What could be more destructive to a man's sense of well-being than the realization that he is becoming sexually dysfunctional? For some men, it is more devastating than learning they have an incurable condition such as cancer. Many reasons account for a man's worry and miserable state of mind. He, of course, misses having satisfying coitus, but the angst includes much more: "I'm no longer virile. I'm losing my manhood. I won't be attractive to my partner. What good is life without sex? What have I done to bring this on? There is probably nothing I can do about it. It will probably get progressively worse."

The man who experiences decreased sexual function and does not feel depressed is a rarity. To make matters worse, the more depressed he becomes, the worse the condition becomes. Also, the feeling of depression interferes with his mental functions so that he is less able to comprehend or deal with the situation.

The man with newly developed sexual shortcomings often tries to put it out of his mind and becomes preoccupied with other interests. This approach often delays or prevents him from seeking help. Usually the man with sexual dysfunction attempts self-treatment by reading material on the subject or talking to a friend. Occasionally this approach is successful. When it isn't, he is even more devastated. It is at this point that he usually seeks medical attention.

It has been clearly shown that when testosterone is administered to those deficient in the hormone, an increased feeling of well-being results. This phenomenon is seen in men of all ages and regardless of the cause for the testosterone deficiency. Research demonstrating this in the elderly is less clear than for younger men. It has been suggested that the benefits of testosterone for those in the older age groups are not as great because of other deteriorating health factors characteristic of the aging process.

For men and their sexual partners, when testosterone deficiency is corrected, the most noticeable and appreciated response is the increase in libido. The men have an increased appetite for sexual activity. Thoughts of sex cross their minds more frequently, and the urge for coitus is more intense. Sexual gratification becomes a stronger motivating force.

If sexual function has declined because of testosterone deficiency, testosterone replacement will have an appreciable and exciting effect (see Chapter 5). Penile erectile function will be restored. The penis becomes more responsive to physical and mental stimuli. The penis during erection is larger and firmer. The duration of the erection is extended. Loss of erection during thrusting is less likely. Muscle weakness and impaired sexual function decrease a man's pleasure in life and his concept of his masculinity. Because of increased muscle strength and endurance when on testosterone, the thrusting is more vigorous and enjoyable. The orgasm is more intense for both the man and his partner. For men who have experienced orgasmic failure, testosterone replacement will decrease the frequency of their failures and often eliminate them.

Testosterone Deficiency and Osteoporosis

Another important condition associated with testosterone deficiency is osteoporosis or bone loss, which can result in frequent bone fractures. Since the 1940s, medical scientists have known that estrogen plays a very important role in the health of women's bones. But not until three decades later did scientists determine that men benefit from the use of testosterone in the same way.

The body needs estrogen or testosterone to maintain healthy, strong bones. Bone composition and structure undergo constant change. Older bone material is steadily lost in a process called *resorption*. At the same time it is constantly replaced with new bone. If the rate of resorption exceeds the rate of replacement, osteoporosis or demineralization occurs. The organic material of bones are cells formed into fibers of a protein substance called *collagen*. This material is impregnated primarily with the two calcium minerals, calcium phosphate (85 percent) and calcium carbonate (10 percent). Other calcium compounds account for the remaining 5 percent.

In osteoporosis, the bones lose calcium and fracture more often and with less severe trauma. Minimal injuries can result in fractures. For example, a fall of only a few inches to a sitting position can fracture the vertebrae. Sharp flexion of the hip or wrist joints can break the bones of these joints. Osteoporosis of the vertebrae may cause chronic pain even when there is no evidence of fracture. The bones most commonly broken are the vertebrae, hips, and wrists.

Deficiencies of estrogen in women and testosterone in men frequently result in osteoporosis, but other causes of this abnormality are possible. An overly active thyroid gland or excessive doses of thyroid medication produce a condition called *thyrotoxicosis,* which is often associated with osteoporosis. Prolonged use of cortisone and related medications also produces osteoporosis, as do poor nutrition and excessive use of alcohol. A common nutritional factor in bone loss is an inadequate intake of calcium.

A prolonged period of bed rest also predictably results in bone loss, and a sedentary lifestyle increases a person's chances of developing osteoporosis. Apparently the effect of gravity influences the metabolism of bone. Astronauts in space for prolonged periods of time, for instance, demonstrate reduced bone mass.

Using estrogen for women to slow the bone destroying process has been recognized as an effective prevention for many years, but the similar benefit of testosterone for men has been slow to catch on. Many studies show that testosterone deficiency accelerates the process of bone demineralization. Medical scientists and clinicians generally agree that testosterone administration retards osteoporosis.

Osteoporosis is the most common bone condition confronting clinicians. Twenty million women demonstrate the condition to a significant degree in the United States, and one million suffer from related fractures. Because men do not have an abrupt total cessation of their sex hormone, the incidence among them is considerably lower—about one and a half million. One-third of the women over age sixty-five will have vertebral fractures. In extreme old age, one in every three women and one in every six men will have hip fractures. By extrapolation, an estimated seven million men over sixty-five will demonstrate osteoporosis. With osteoporosis resulting in fractures, the consequences are just as severe for men as for women.

Because osteoporosis and the related fractures occur in later life, these fractures are more serious, debilitating, and threatening. Many in the older age groups also have other potentially dangerous illnesses, such as diabetes, lung disease, and heart disease. These may be well tolerated and managed until an additional insult is added, such as a disabling fracture. An osteoporotic fracture can tip the scales. A major surgery to pin a hip or a confinement to bed or a wheelchair adds to the stress of the preexisting conditions. Permanent disability or even death may ensue.

Middle-aged women who have suffered major bouts of depression have significantly weaker bones than other women in their age group, and they may run risk of fractures. Depressed women's bone mineral density is 6 percent lower on average in the spine and 10 to 14 percent lower in the hip, a level of bone loss equivalent to postmenopausal osteoporosis, but in women whose average age is only forty-one. One hypothesis from researchers is that depression affects hormone secretions. No similar study has yet been done for men, but because of the hormonal parallels in men and women affecting osteoporosis and depression, there is certainly a possibility that clinically depressed men might also suffer from bone loss.

Testosterone Deficiency and Depression

For decades, mental health professionals have used the word *depression* to designate a mood or affective disorder. Clinical or major depression is a mental disorder and not the same as a sadness or dejection that is typical of grieving or unhappiness. Clinical depression is believed to be a chemical abnormality that occurs at the connections of brain cells. In addition to unhappiness, symptoms of chemical depression include a low energy level, poor self-esteem, and feelings of helplessness or hopelessness. People experiencing clinical depression often have changes in eating and sleeping habits. Antidepressant medications can correct this chemical defect.

Unhappiness, grieving, and similar dysphoria respond to psychological counseling but are not responsive to antidepressant medications. Some television shows and magazine articles promote testosterone as a treatment for depression. They suggest the hormone is a panacea for any unhappiness men might experience. No medical evidence indicates that testosterone reduces dysphoria, regardless of the cause. The truth regarding benefits of testosterone for depression lies somewhere in between. Testosterone can be used to indirectly treat the dysphoria that results from testosterone deficiency, but it is totally useless in the treatment of clinical depression.

Between the times when a man recognizes a sexual disorder and his first visit to his physician, he will undoubtedly experience a feeling of depression. With appropriate investigation and treatment, the symptoms are lessened and the unhappiness dwindles away. If the cause of his condition is testosterone deficiency and it is successfully treated, he no longer feels depressed. So it can be said that testosterone therapy removed his depression, even though it happens indirectly.

It has been scientifically proven that testosterone replacement reestablishes a feeling of well-being. It restores a man's sense of joy and contentment. The improvement in physical vigor is a big boost to a man's morale. The rejuvenating effect on his sexuality replaces worry and unhappiness with self-confidence and pleasure. For the clinically depressed, testosterone is of no benefit. It does not replace antidepressant medication, but testosterone is recommended for those men who have both clinical depression and testosterone deficiency.

Though no indisputable scientific evidence suggests that men with testosterone deficiency are happier when treated with the hormone, most physicians treating the condition are confident that their patients are much more energetic and more contented when treated. It is unlikely that testosterone elevates mood when administered to those who are not testosterone deficient.

Because multiple benefits from prescribing testosterone accrue for those with a deficiency of the hormone, a few health providers administer testosterone to those who have some of the symptoms of the deficiency but are not actually deficient. The providers and their patients believe, or at least hope, testosterone will have magical effects on sexual performance and will produce a feeling of well-being. It is hoped that future research will clarify the relationship between testosterone use and the psychological symptoms men experience that are not due to a demonstrable testosterone deficiency.

Testosterone Deficiency and Changes in Memory and Cognition

Does testosterone improve the memory of a man who is deficient in the hormone? Does it improve his cognition or his capacity to perceive, think, reflect, ponder, meditate? The medical research on estrogen for women is far ahead of that on testosterone for men. Studies show that menopausal women have improved memory and cognition when receiving estrogen. Some medical scientists and clinicians believe testosterone will similarly improve memory and cognition in men who have testosterone deficiency. Early investigation on animals seems to support this theory.

Basic neurological investigations show the brain has estrogen receptors, that is, molecular structures in the brain cells or cell membranes that bind to estrogen. Evidence of testosterone receptors in the brain is as yet sketchy or nonexistent. Many anecdotal reports claim that testosterone improves the function of men's minds, but these are not substantiated by scientific investigation. Nevertheless, some health providers promote testosterone to patients for improving cognition without proof. It is not yet known whether this apparent benefit is due to a placebo effect. It should be remembered that many, many factors influence the workings of the mind. Several clinicians and researchers expect that, in the future, testosterone will prove to be effective for improving memory and cognition for men, just as estrogen has for women.

CHAPTER FIVE

Back to the Good Life

Testosterone Replacement Therapy

- **Advantages of TRT: Overview**
- **Advantages of TRT: Sexual Functioning**
- **Other Health Benefits**

- **Methods of Administration**
- **Length of Treatment**
- **Side Effects**
- **Prognosis**

any deficiency diseases exist, and the treatment for most of them is replacement therapy. Correction of testosterone deficiency is just as important for the medical care for men as is the administration of insulin for diabetics or thyroid hormone for patients with hypothyroid conditions. Testosterone replacement treatment (TRT) improves sexual functioning and increases muscle strength and endurance. The masculine characteristics of a man's physique are enhanced. Correction of the deficiency restores a man's libido, vigor, and energy, and his mental attitude improves as he becomes aware of his physical restoration.

Medical science is entering a new era in understanding and treating testosterone deficiency, however the research and knowledge about it are comparable to where estrogen deficiency research was fifty years ago. The underlying cause of both estrogen deficiency and testosterone deficiency is the same—gonadal failure that leads to a decrease in the amount of sex hormones. In women the ovaries stop producing sufficient estrogen, and in men the testes no longer create sufficient testosterone. The failures are irreversible except in rare cases.

Both men and women suffer the mental and physical changes of decreasing sex hormone production in their bodies. The symptoms are somewhat dissimilar, but untreated, the prognosis is equally unfavorable. There are significant differences in the prognosis for men and women when they develop deficiencies in their sex hormones, but the recovery with replacement therapy is quite similar: both men and women have an improved prognosis.

Fortunately, testosterone deficiency is totally reversible. Nowadays no man has to suffer the insults of hormonal deficiency to his psyche or his body. Men whose gonads produce inadequate amounts of testosterone are able to receive the hormone from external sources. Testosterone can be introduced into his body and have the same effect as that produced by the body itself. The chemical is exactly the same whether from an external or internal source.

Until 1935, testosterone was obtained by extraction from mammalian gonads. Since then the product has been synthetically produced in the laboratory and manufacturing facilities by chemical manipulation of other substances such as cholesterol. For practical reasons such as ease and cost, testosterone is no longer obtained from natural sources.

Testosterone is the only male sex hormone approved for treating the deficiency by the Food and Drug Administration (FDA). Many other hormonal products such as DHEA are not approved by the FDA (see the Appendix and Chapter 3 for a discussion of DHEA). These other products are sold over the counter, but only by mislabeling them as dietary supplements can they bypass federal regulations. Imitator drugs such as those promoted as age retardants, sex stimulants, and muscle builders are uncontrolled, and production and labeling standards have not been established. There is no way for the buyer to know which product is safe, what dosage gives the best results (if any), and what their side effects and long-term effects are.

Until recently, most physicians only prescribed testosterone replacement therapy for men diagnosed with hypogonadism, a condition in which the testicles produce inadequate testosterone. It is now becoming more common to prescribe TRT for men who have low testosterone levels or symptoms of testosterone deficiency as a result of the natural aging process even if they don't fit the precise definition for testosterone deficiency.

A man who is considering TRT needs to be able to evaluate whether using supplemental testosterone is right for him. In addition to the benefits that TRT offers, a number of other factors to consider include cost, convenience, and the potential side effects.

Advantages of TRT: Overview

The symptoms of testosterone deficiency, as described in Chapter 4, can include a decrease in a man's overall sense of well-being, less productivity, feeling less masculine and less aggressive, loss in muscle strength, depression, lowered self-esteem, and a reduced sex drive. If a true deficiency exists, taking supplemental testosterone can improve or reverse all of these symptoms.

The most immediate and obvious benefit of TRT is an improvement in mood and an enhanced sense of well-being. Mood elevation is one of the main reasons testosterone-treated men believe testosterone to be an antiaging drug. Nearly every medical textbook, as well as articles in the medical literature on the subject, confirms there is a heightened feeling of well-being when testosterone is used. Some patients refer to this as a "testosterone high." The good feeling is reminiscent of how they felt in their younger years. They are aware of a boost in their energy level. The work they do is less tiring, and they like the feeling of greater endurance. A man who feels good is better able to enjoy all aspects of his life—family, work, recreation. Personal relationships are improved. Family and associates see the man as rejuvenated. A sense of well-being increases the ability to handle disappointments and problems in life appropriately.

There is considerable variation in the time before patients are aware of the heightened mood. It may be four to eight days before this change becomes readily apparent. The change is gradual, and sometimes a spouse or close friend will notice it before the patient himself does.

Complementing the rise in mood is a rise in overall energy. Better mood and energy may translate into a greater competitive edge in professional matters, which can increase a man's productivity. The sense of satisfaction in, and enjoyment of, his work returns.

Another early change that men experience is an increase in their libido. Some scientific evidence indicates that healthy people (men and women) have enhanced libido regardless of their innate testosterone levels when given the hormone. The heightened urge for sexual activity occurs within two or three days of an injection and within a week or two with patches.

Muscle changes are the last to appear. Tape measurements are somewhat unreliable, but men are fairly sensitive to changes in how their clothing fits. Some men report smaller belt sizes; some report that the androgen reduces abdominal fat deposits. Reliable evidence also suggests that supplementary testosterone increases the size and strength of muscles, but the bulk of this evidence is based on studies of the anabolic steroids. This response is not completely understood, but the anaerobic effects of androgens is well documented. For the last four decades physicians have been using testosterone and modified androgens to assist chronically ill patients to build stronger bodies and improve metabolic activity.

Advantages of TRT: Sexual Functioning

The most noticeable and appreciated response to TRT is the rise in libido. A man experiences a greater appetite for sexual activity. The number of erections occurring weekly increases. Visual, auditory, and tactile senses are more sensitive. He gets more pleasure from observing his partner's appearance and actions. Masturbation provides more pleasure. Thoughts of sex cross his mind more frequently, and the urge for coitus occurs more often and more intensely. Sexual gratification becomes a stronger motivating force.

If there has been impaired sexual function due to testosterone deficiency, testosterone replacement will have an appreciable and exciting effect. Penile erectile function is restored. The penis becomes more responsive to both physical and mental stimuli. The penis during erection is larger and firmer. Although there is no increase in the circumference of the erect penis, the maximum level of rigidity increases. Nocturnal erections occur more frequently, and the duration of the erection is extended. Loss of erection during thrusting is less likely. Because of increased muscle strength and endurance, the thrusting tends to be more vigorous and enjoyable. The orgasm is more intense for both the man and his partner. For men who have experienced orgasmic failure, testosterone will decrease the frequency of the failures and often eliminates them entirely.

Other Health Benefits

A number of nonsexual physical health benefits for men on testosterone replacement therapy also occur. The muscles regain some of their strength and mass when there is more testosterone circulating. The basal (baseline) metabolic rate increases significantly with TRT, which signifies an improvement in metabolism. While body weight increases, lean body mass also goes up, with less visceral fat mass or body fat. In many normal, healthy men, one sign of encroaching middle age is the development of a stomach paunch. A study showed that middle-aged men who used testosterone skin patches for nine months benefited as indicated by a significant decline in their abdominal fat accompanied by general metabolic and circulatory improvements.

In addition, with TRT less calcium is excreted in the urine, which means the bones stay stronger and are more resistant to osteoporosis. This result is significant because one and a half million men in the United States have osteoporosis. Testosterone does not reverse osteoporosis, but it does retard the process. It is reported that osteoporosis and resulting fractures occur in men with gonadal insufficiency, so early recognition and replacement therapy for testosterone deficiency are of definite value.

The risk of heart disease is lower because total cholesterol levels go down as well as the harmful low-density lipoprotein (LDL) cholesterol levels. Diastolic blood pressure also decreases. The hematocrit (red blood cell count) increases, which improves the blood's capacity to carry oxygen. The more oxygen that reaches the tissues, the more efficiently they function.

A man on TRT also develops better resistance to diabetes because the amount of glucose in the blood goes down and insulin resistance improves.

Methods of Administration

Until the testosterone patches became available, testosterone was administered in daily ten- to fifty-milligram methyltestosterone tablets to swallow, buccal (cheek) tablets, sublingual (under the tongue) tablets, and injections.

Testosterone Tablets

Testosterone is available in tablet form for swallowing. After the tablets are absorbed into the bloodstream, the hormone goes directly to the liver. Here, much of the hormone is changed into inactive chemicals that do not produce the desired effects in the body. These inactive substances are excreted, which obviously presents a problem in trying to achieve the desired effect. (This is an even greater problem for testosterone therapy than for estrogen therapy.)

Buccal tablets, five to twenty-five milligrams a day, are placed against the inside of the cheek and left there to dissolve. The hormone absorbs through the mucus membrane into the bloodstream, bypassing the liver and avoiding the first pass-through. This delivery system has never gained popularity among physicians or their patients because the degree of absorption is variable so it cannot be depended on to achieve the desired effect. It must be used several times each day, and patients find it inconvenient. The same drawbacks apply to sublingual tablets, which are placed under the tongue, held there, and allowed to absorb.

Testosterone Injections

Testosterone by injection has been the most widely used method of administration. Injections are effective because the absorption is predictable. Also, most of the early liver destruction is avoided with shots.

Injectable testosterone is available in two basic forms, short- and long-acting. Ten to fifty milligrams of the short-acting type is administered two or three times a week, and fifty to four hundred milligrams of the long-acting form at two- to four-week intervals. Long-acting injections are usually injected into deep-muscle tissue, such as the buttocks, and don't begin to act until two or three days later.

Like tablets, injections also entail some inconvenience. Many men do not like receiving shots or have trouble fitting appointments for them into their weekly schedule. A disadvantage of the long-acting injection is the gradual loss of effectiveness over the two- or three-week interval. This loss is minor and of no clinical significance the first week or so, but it becomes significant and detectable by the patient the last week of a three-week schedule. For this reason, many patients choose to have the injections every two rather than three weeks even though it is less convenient.

Some men believe they can feel their testosterone blood level becoming too low a few days before they are due for their next injection. A minority of men avoid injections because they dislike needles, but most lose that fear over time. With injections, a small percentage of men report a brief period of pain at the site of the injection. Home injections of testosterone are a less expensive and satisfactory solution if someone is available who has been properly taught and is confident about skillfully giving the injection. In many cases, a man's partner may give the injections. Women tend to be less squeamish about needles, and they may find giving the shots easy and be pleased to participate in their partner's care. After the first injection or two, the man develops confidence in his partner's skill and is appreciative.

Testosterone Patches

Patches can be used to deliver substances into the body. As the substance comes in contact with the skin, it is absorbed through the skin and taken up by the circulatory system. Some substances are absorbed well, some not at all, and for others absorption is somewhere in between. The popular scopolamine patch ocean travelers wear behind the ear to prevent sea sickness is an example of fairly good skin absorption. Both the male and female sex hormones are well absorbed through the skin, and estrogen has been used in skin patches for several years. In June 1994, the first practical means of testosterone administration via patches became available in the United States.

The testosterone skin patch delivers the testosterone into the circulation more effectively and conveniently than previously prescribed methods. The first patch introduced, Testoderm, is worn on the scrotum. The scrotal skin is thinner than the skin of the trunk and extremities and is more permeable. It does not require an additional substance to enhance absorption. Before application, the scrotal skin is shaved to improve adherence of the patch. Wearing briefs rather than boxer-style underwear also improves adherence. The primary disadvantage of applying the patch to the scrotum is that the scrotal patch adheres better when the scrotum is shaved and the patch is preheated with a hair dryer.

Testoderm contains ten to fifteen milligrams of testosterone and delivers four or six milligrams of testosterone a day. A new patch, applied in the morning, must be changed every twenty-two to twenty-four hours to be effective.

The second patch, Androderm, is placed on skin other than the scrotum, using a total of two patches. The recommended sites are the abdomen, back, chest, shin, thigh, and upper arm. The most consistent testosterone input occurs when the patch is on the back, thigh, upper arm, or abdomen, and these are considered the optimal placement sites. The nonscrotal patches are changed once daily at bedtime. After a period of therapy, if blood tests indicate two patches are more than needed, a reduction to one patch daily may be appropriate. If two patches do not elevate the testosterone to the desired level, a third, nonscrotal patch is added. Some recent research has shown that using one nonscrotal patches can be just as effective as two.

Testosterone patches are just as effective as injections because they increase the blood levels of testosterone in the same way. However, it is simpler to regulate the blood levels using injections because they can be fine-tuned by altering the dose injected or the time interval between injections. One promotional point the manufacturers make about the patches is that users do not have the high and low effects that come with the injections; the testosterone delivery is more consistent. The timing of patch application more closely simulates the normal circadian pattern of the body's testosterone levels.

The cost differs significantly between testosterone patches and injections. The long-lasting injections can cost as little as $8 a month, and the shorter-duration injections about $50 a month. Currently the two main brands of patches being used cost about $80 to $100 a month.

Some men find applying a new patch every day inconvenient, and 13 to 37 percent of patch users experience some skin reaction to the patch's adhesive (similar to the reaction some people have to the adhesive in surgical tape or bandages). The reaction is usually limited to local irritation and redness and is seldom severe. About one man in twenty discontinues the patches because of the irritation. Blistering is rare, occurring in only about one in every six thousand applications.

Length of Treatment

The duration of testosterone replacement depends on how long a person wants to continue receiving the benefits of the sex hormone. The deteriorating effects of the deficiency return soon after TRT is discontinued. Very few causes of low levels of testosterone are reversible, either medically or surgically, so once the need is present, the hormone is usually continued permanently with occasional dose modifications. As long as a man wishes to enjoy the benefits of replacement therapy or have protection against the bone fractures of osteoporosis, he must continue the long-term therapy.

If a man wishes to discontinue the therapy because of cost, inconvenience, or other personal reasons, the testosterone may be withdrawn abruptly. No withdrawal symptoms result except for the return of the previous deficiency symptoms. When testosterone is discontinued, there is a gradual increase in the rate at which the bones' demineralization occurs. With or without testosterone therapy, this rate of loss is also affected by calcium intake and exercise. Use of some drugs—for example, the corticosteroids—increases the rate of bone mineral loss.

One exception to continuing TRT is if prostate cancer is present. Most clinicians advise the withdrawal of testosterone if they diagnose a prostatic malignancy. New research shows that a cycle of testosterone blocking and testosterone administration can keep prostate cancer in check for many years. Testosterone appears to alternately feed and suppress cancer growth over the long term. In 80 percent of patients treated with antitestosterone therapy—either removing the testes or using a chemical that blocks the action of the hormone—the cancer almost always returns within one to three years because the cancer cells learn to grow in the absence of testosterone and become sensitized to it. When they do, administering small amounts of testosterone can kill the cancer cells.

Both injection and patch users require regular monitoring and testing of their cholesterol and PSA (prostate-specific antigen, screened to determine the presence or absence of prostate cancer) levels for as long as they are receiving TRT (the relationship between TRT and prostate cancer is discussed later in this chapter and also in Chapter 8). The screening procedure for the PSA and cholesterol profile is the same for patch users as for men who receive injected testosterone. Part of the monitoring regimen for men using TRT is blood tests to check testosterone levels. Not all physicians agree as to how frequently this testing should be done. Early in treatment the tests are performed more often to assist in adjusting the dose, usually every three to four weeks. After the adjustment period, the tests are done every three months and eventually at six-month intervals.

Side Effects

In the short term, absolutely no undesirable side effects result from testosterone replacement therapy. When one remembers that it is a supplement to a natural hormone already in the body, this fact is understandable. The common side effects from most drugs occur in the gastrointestinal system: nausea, vomiting, abdominal discomfort, diarrhea, and constipation. These disturbances occur less often with testosterone patches, injections, and buccal tablets than with oral tablets because the stomach and intestinal tract are bypassed by the first three delivery methods. Occasionally a man may have an allergic reaction to taking testosterone (such as a rash similar to those that can occur when beginning any new food or medication), but less than 1 percent of men do (such an allergy is different than possible irritation at the patch site due to the adhesive).

These allergic symptoms will subside after the drug is discontinued. With the possible exception of the effect of testosterone on the prostate, the side effects are very rarely significant and don't require discontinuing TRT. Seldom do men find the side effects troublesome enough to stop using the hormone, but a man's physician has the responsibility to assist him in making that decision.

For the majority of men, the only negative aspects of testosterone therapy are inconvenience, cost, and the need for scheduled lab tests and monitoring, although there are a few potential long-term side effects from TRT. These include a slightly lowered high-density lipoprotein (HDL, or "good") cholesterol level, edema (water retention), jaundice when taking testosterone orally, gynecomastia (enlargement and tenderness of the breasts) that resolves with continued treatment, acne, and benign prostate enlargement (also known as benign prostatic hyperplasia, or BPH). If benign prostate enlargement occurs in a man taking testosterone therapy, his physician must determine whether it's a usual and expected change consistent with age or whether the hormone is a contributing factor. The physician must then decide, taking into account the patient's preference, whether the change in the prostate size warrants stopping TRT.

Benign prostate enlargement is under the control of dihydrotestosterone, the active form of testosterone. The prostate surrounds the urethra as it leaves the bladder. When the gland enlarges, it encroaches on the urethra and affects urination. When this happens, the urinary stream is decreased in caliber and has less force. An enlarged prostate interferes with complete bladder emptying; consequently, the bladder fills sooner and has to be emptied more often, which is especially annoying at night when it disturbs sleep. In the rare case when the condition occurs during TRT, the testosterone is usually discontinued. If BPH continues to be a problem after the testosterone administration is stopped, the doctor may prescribe a medication that reduces the obstruction. Whenever testosterone is administered, the patient's response and side effects are monitored regularly.

Testosterone replacement therapy can induce raised PSA levels, and whether it's justified or not, prostate cancer becomes of concern. For many years clinicians have questioned the possibility of testosterone causing the prostate malignancy, although no reliable scientific research indicates a causal relationship. The issue is confusing because it is known that if a prostate cancer already exists, testosterone makes it grow faster and spread more. This is the primary reason for regular monitoring by PSA blood tests and digital prostate examinations. If a malignancy is suspected, the testosterone is withdrawn and additional studies are performed to determine whether a cancer exists. The effect of testosterone on prostate cancer is the main argument against prescribing TRT unless there is a definite deficiency with symptoms serious enough to indicate a need for using the hormone. (This issue is analogous to the question of whether the female hormone estrogen causes breast cancer in women.)

Estrogen is used, though rarely, in men to slow the growth and spread of prostate cancer. The female hormone counteracts the testosterone effect of increasing the cancer growth when administered to men with advanced prostate cancer.

Prognosis

The prognosis for a man with testosterone deficiency is progressively unfavorable unless therapy is instituted. He gradually becomes less virile. He becomes less vigorous and energetic. He loses his muscle strength and suffers a reduction in his sexuality. As the level of testosterone decreases, mineral loss from the bones accelerates, which poses a greater risk for fractures. This prognosis remains unfavorable unless the deficiency is corrected.

The prognosis is excellent for the testosterone-deficient man who receives hormone replacement. In adequate doses, regardless of the route of administration, testosterone prevents the symptoms of depression, listlessness, and loss of energy. It also helps maintain strong bones. Testosterone replacement restores a man's sexual capabilities to the same level as a man of the same age whose gonads are producing adequate testosterone. The sex hormones retard some of the characteristic changes of aging so that the man on hormone replacement therapy has, in some ways, a better prognosis than the man who experiences the normal gonadal diminution of testosterone production.

CHAPTER SIX

Robert

A Case History
of Testosterone Deficiency

T his chapter reviews the actual medical record of a middle-aged man who visited his doctor because he was unhappy and didn't know why. At his wife's urging, he came to my office for a physical examination, which revealed that he was suffering from a testosterone deficiency.

This chapter describes a typical medical history, physical examination, laboratory tests, diagnosis, and treatment. The case has a happy ending. With treatment, the patient has become a much happier man. His relationships have improved, he has become more productive, he's healthier and stronger, his muscle size has increased, and his libido and sexuality have been restored.

An Oregon rain was falling, and the morning was gloomy. Robert's mood matched the weather. When I greeted him in the reception room, his manner was somewhat unfriendly. I invited him to have a seat in the consultation room, and he slumped into the chair.

My effort to exchange pleasantries was futile, so I started taking Robert's medical history. "What is your chief symptom?" I asked.

His answer didn't surprise me, considering his mood. "I don't have any symptoms. I'm only here because Beth insisted. I'm fine, but she thinks I must be sick because I act differently."

"Do you think you act differently?"

A trace of anger crossed his face. "No, but she thinks I'm less fun to live with. It seems to me that we just have less to talk about."

I had known Robert and Beth both as personal acquaintances and patients for twenty-two years and had delivered their youngest child. Robert was sixty-three, and Beth was fifty-seven. Five months earlier they had bought a new house in town. The three older children were married and had homes of their own. The youngest was in college. A year after her daughter started college, Beth had found a job in one of the local banks. She was apparently a good employee and very much enjoyed her work. With the change in her lifestyle, she had seemed to take on a new personality. She now had a sense of independence and self-confidence that hadn't been previously apparent.

Robert was a fellow member of a service club to which I belonged. He had always been pleasant and somewhat jovial until the past the eighteen months, when his manner had turned somewhat subdued. Now at the lunch meetings he contributed very little to the table conversation. On a recent office visit for a respiratory infection, he had even appeared a bit testy.

While taking his medical history, I found he had good health habits, including a balanced diet, regular exercise, and adequate rest. He had started smoking cigarettes when he was sixteen and had smoked an average of one pack a day except for four years while in the service, when he averaged two packs a day. He had managed to quit two years previously at age sixty-one when his brother, who also smoked, was diagnosed with lung cancer. There was nothing to suggest cardiovascular or gastrointestinal disease, but the genitourinary history revealed two significant symptoms. During the previous two years, he had been annoyed by waking up in the middle of the night to empty his bladder. This disruption was especially troublesome because he was unable to return to sleep promptly. While lying awake he was troubled by perceived problems such as financial and retirement concerns.

After the routine medical history was finished, Robert became more relaxed and willing to talk about the reason for the office visit—Beth's observation that he was "acting differently." I asked a few leading questions about behavioral changes he might be aware of himself. He soon became introspective and started unloading.

He first described what he considered to be his physical symptoms. About two years previously he became aware of a reduced energy level, which he described by saying, "I had less pep." He then enumerated some observations about himself. "I am slow getting started in the mornings. It takes more coffee to get up to speed. I have to push myself to get going on tasks. I put less energy and enthusiasm in the sales meetings I conduct. I don't seem to get revved up about my golf game the way I used to."

Robert felt slightly fatigued all day long, not just in the late afternoons and evenings. He hated to get up in the morning and mildly dreaded going to work. At work he was bored and found his job less interesting than in the past. He observed a reduction in his innovative skills and aggressive nature. These changes made him a little irritable because he had always taken pride in his work. His drive was apparently part of his self-image, so the comments he was hearing from his family, clients, and friends about his lessened productivity angered him.

The reduced energy level intruded in his personal life in several ways. He had lost some of his interest in home and friends. This attitude shift probably was what Beth meant when she said that he was "less fun to live with." In the past he had enjoyed visiting friends and entertaining them in his home. These diversions now were drudgery. He had lost his imagination for finding fun and exciting things to do. He disliked planning parties and other social events.

As Robert described these changes, I began wondering whether he had slipped into a depression. After inquiring about other symptoms that might suggest such a diagnosis, it seemed unlikely, but I still listed depression in his chart as a possible explanation for the symptoms.

When I asked Robert about his sexual function, he answered, "Oh, yeah, it's OK." But when I asked about specifics, it became apparent that it really wasn't OK. His libido had decreased rather abruptly, starting three years before. He thought about sex, but it was usually in response to stimuli, such as seeing an R-rated movie or provocative pictures or reading erotic fiction.

When Robert was a teenager, sex was on his mind much of the time, as it is with most teens, and he masturbated frequently, some days as many as six times. He lost his virginity in his twenties and spent considerable time and effort developing his sexual relationships with women.

Robert and Beth were married when he was thirty-six and she was twenty-nine. Beth was still a virgin when they wed. After some of the usual minor sexual adjustment problems during the first four months of marriage, their sexual activity became vigorous and frequent. They physically expressed their love for each other through coitus six to twelve times a week. Their first child was born two and a half years after the marriage. During the childbearing and rearing years, Beth became less sexual, and the frequency of their sexual intercourse decreased to two or three times a week. The reduced amount of sexual activity was acceptable to Robert. During these years he was physically and mentally occupied with his business. He had purchased an insurance agency and his work was very demanding, requiring evening hours and trips out of town.

Beth's interest in sex increased significantly after their last child moved out to go to college. Although Beth was never demanding, Robert sensed that more sexual encounters would have pleased her. It surprised him when she started showing an interest in pornographic movies and novels. He was pleased, but slightly dismayed, by her interest in experimentation with different sexual techniques.

Robert was aware that his sexual appetite had been waning during the previous five years, but it had only been during the last six months that the reduced libido bothered him. He recalled having an almost constant need for sex in his younger years, and when he made the comparison with his current libido, the difference left him feeling depressed. As it is for most men, his self-image was closely related to his perceived sexual prowess. He disliked the thought of aging as much as anyone else does.

Robert's awareness of Beth's increased libido also concerned him because he deeply loved his wife and wanted her to be happy. His belief that she would like to have coitus more often (and that she would be a happier person if she did) was depressing. Even though he was confident of Beth's love for him, he had fleeting fears that she might be tempted to enter an extramarital relationship. Such thoughts arose rarely but were very disquieting when they did. His fear was more likely to occur when the couple were together around people, for example, at parties. He would notice his wife's seemingly unusual interest in and conversation with another man. After such a party, he would become impatient with Beth. He would realize the next day, when recalling the events of the evening, that his thoughts had been irrational and his behavior inappropriate. He usually gave himself an excuse by blaming the amount of alcohol he had consumed. His irritability at these times partially contributed to Beth's assessment of his "acting differently."

The rest of Robert's genitourinary history was also significant. For the past year his erectile function had diminished. Occasionally he would experience a delay in developing an adequate erection for intromission (insertion of the penis into the vagina), but he rarely had a complete failure. Robert was more disturbed when he lost his erection while thrusting after intromission, although he was not overly worried because the loss of erection usually occurred when he was particularly tired or had drunk an excessive amount of alcohol.

I didn't detect any significant abnormalities during Robert's physical examination. His blood pressure was in the high-normal range, and he was slightly overweight, but otherwise the physical findings were consistent with those of a healthy man his age. His prostate gland was not enlarged, there were no nodules in his prostate, and its firmness was even throughout. The testes were of normal size, and no soft-ness or abnormal tenderness was evident. One testis was 20 percent larger than the other, but not a significant variation in most men.

After the examination, I reported to Robert that his heart, lungs, abdomen, genitals, and prostate were all normal. I then briefly discussed with him some of the possible condi-tions that might explain the behavioral changes he and his wife had observed. The possibilities included abnormal thyroid function, diabetes, gonad insufficiency, and other endocrine (glandular) disorders.

A nurse drew a blood sample and had Robert leave a urine specimen for various laboratory tests. Robert scheduled another office visit to discuss the results of the tests, diagnosis, and management of his symptoms of irritability, reduced energy level, and sexuality changes.

Beth accompanied Robert when he returned to get his laboratory reports. Even though I had asked him to bring her with him for the visit, I was surprised to see her. Men seldom are willing to bring their partners with them to a consultation. Either they discourage their partner's presence or just don't let their partners know I've requested it. There may be several reasons that the patient chooses to not have a partner present for the reports and diagnosis. A common one is the fear of being told of a chronic, severe, or even fatal condition they would not want their partners to learn about in a doctor's office. Nevertheless, a consultation is usually more productive if the spouse is present, so I appreciated Beth's coming and I told them this when they arrived.

I started by reading to them the record of the medical history I had taken. This serves two purposes. First, the patient has a chance to correct the record or add to it if he wishes. Robert agreed I had correctly dictated the history and he had nothing to add. The second purpose is to let the partner know what transpired at the first visit and to add her own observations.

Beth had nothing to add but confirmed, emphatically, Robert's symptoms. I told Beth that Robert's physical examination had been normal and provided no explanations for the symptoms. Next, I presented the laboratory results and their significance.

The urinalysis was normal, as were most of the blood tests. The blood sugar and thyroid stimulating hormone (TSH) levels were normal, so diabetes and thyroid disease were ruled out. Normal levels of various body chemicals—potassium, sodium, chloride, calcium, phosphorous—helped eliminate some other diseases. Serum iron level, normal hemoglobin, and the red blood cell count ruled out such conditions as anemia. The liver and kidney tests were also within normal limits.

Robert's blood cholesterol and other lipid levels were slightly unfavorable, but not enough to explain any of the symptoms. Because high blood cholesterol and lipid levels can produce long-term negative effects on the arteries, I suggested some dietary modifications. When discussing diet with a man, it is helpful to have his partner present so that they can prepare nutritious meals together. I reserved the discussion of the results of the testosterone blood test for last since the results were significant. Robert's testosterone level was abnormally low at 208 nanograms per deciliter. The normal level for Robert's age group is 300 to 1,000 nanograms per deciliter.

Naturally, Robert and Beth wanted to know whether there was a cure for testosterone deficiency. I told them that no cure exists but fortunately the condition is controllable. As with most deficiency diseases, the treatment consists of replacing the chemical the body is missing. There are many examples of this kind of treatment: insulin for diabetes, thyroid extract for hypothyroidism, and estrogen for menopause.

I listed the present-day forms of testosterone administration that were available and evaluated the advantages and disadvantages of each, including effectiveness, side effects, convenience of administration, and cost (see Chapter 5). I covered the short- and long-term benefits of testosterone replacement—elimination of symptoms and protection of bones against fractures in later life (see Chapter 4).

Robert had a number of options to consider: whether to accept or reject the diagnosis and, if he accepted it, whether to treat the deficiency and which form of testosterone to use. I encouraged him to go home and discuss the options with Beth and not to make an immediate decision. I've learned through years of practice that there are advantages to giving patients adequate time to consider new diagnoses and treatment options before starting a new regimen. Otherwise, some patients feel they have been pressured. Because of anxiety associated with a visit to the doctor's office and hearing the diagnosis and treatment, some patients do not remember or assimilate the information completely. They often need a return visit to ask questions before deciding about treatment. Consideration of treatment is especially important when it's a lifetime commitment being considered, as in Robert's case. This approach is not because stopping the medication might be fatal but because if it is beneficial and improves the patient's health, he will want to continue the medication indefinitely.

At my suggestion, Robert arranged for another appointment a few days later, and I encouraged Beth to be present again. As Robert left, I gave him some reading material on the subject of testosterone deficiency to study at home.

During the next visit, I asked whether he had any questions, and he indicated he didn't but was a bit apprehensive about testosterone's effect on the prostate. He had read a magazine article that suggested testosterone may cause prostate cancer. I explained the relationship between testosterone and prostate cancer thoroughly for him (see Chapter 5). Robert indicated that he was willing to accept the possible risks of testosterone replacement therapy to have the benefits. He chose regular, long-term injection as the route of administration. I suggested that after two or three injections in the office, he might want to bring Beth so that she could learn how to give him the shots. The nurse gave the first injection, and an appointment was made for the next one three weeks later. I told the receptionist to allow time for a brief office visit at the time of the next injection, because most patients think of some questions after the first injection. Appointments were also made for several weeks later to run another testosterone blood level test and an office visit to follow after the test results were available.

During the first follow-up visit, preceding the second injection, Robert expressed mild disappointment, saying he felt no different but was pleased with the increase he noticed in his libido. I explained that, although improved libido may begin early in the treatment, the more subtle responses take considerably longer. Both Robert and his wife definitely wanted to continue the hormone replacement therapy. Robert had noticed no unfavorable side effects, so the second injection was given.

About ten weeks after starting therapy and after three injections, Robert's blood was drawn to determine his testosterone level. An appointment to report the results was made for the following week, and Robert was asked to bring Beth to that appointment.

On arrival, they both appeared to be in a happy mood. They reported that their sexual activity had increased in frequency to about twice a week. They expressed the hope that the injections would continue. I reported that the level of testosterone in Robert's blood had elevated and was now in the middle of the normal reference range. It was almost twice that of the preliminary level. The three of us agreed to continue the injections every two weeks and that Beth would take over administering the shots.

Beth participated in a brief training session. The nurse explained to her the basics of intramuscular injections, including how to load the syringe and maintain sterility. Beth then watched the nurse preparing and filling the syringe, inserting the needle into Robert's buttock, and pressing the plunger to deposit the testosterone deep into the muscle. Beth seemed satisfied that she could do the injection without difficulty. An appointment was made for two weeks later when Beth would do the injection under the nurse's supervision.

When they returned for the appointment, Beth was eager to give the shot and said, "I'm ready to do my thing." Robert seemed only slightly apprehensive. Afterward it was obvious that Beth was pleased with her own performance and that Robert was somewhat relieved when he said, "She's a good nurse—I hardly felt it." I gave Robert prescriptions for a vial of testosterone, syringes, and needles and asked them to call if either of them had any problems or questions regarding home administration of the medication.

Robert's testosterone blood level was satisfactory at his six-month check-up, and he was satisfied with the results of the injections. His sexuality had been restored, and, just as important, his mood had improved. His energy level was up, which he felt was improving his work productivity. He added, "Everything is better at home, too." The prostate-specific antigen (PSA) of the blood was unchanged from the first determination, and the examination of his prostate was negative for any evidence of cancer.

Robert's blood tests and physical examination were still normal at his first yearly visit. We agreed to continue the testosterone replacement therapy, and I gave him the option of using testosterone patches. He chose to continue having his wife give him the injections at two-week intervals.

Several years later, Robert remains happy and healthy. His tests for prostate cancer are negative, and he demonstrates no unfavorable side effects from the testosterone. Robert's case history is fairly typical of testosterone deficiency and a positive response to therapy.

CHAPTER SEVEN

Midlife Crises

Testosterone Deficiency and "Male Menopause"

- **The Causes of Andropause**
- **Testosterone Deficiency and Andropause**

he term *male menopause* is widely used when referring to an unhappy stage of a man's life. This term was probably popularized because the condition occurs at the same time in a man's life that women experience menopause. *Andropause* ("male menopause") and menopause do have some psychological symptoms in common. However, *menopause* is not an appropriate word to apply to men because it specifically refers to the cessation of menstruation in the human female. During the past decade, the trend has been to refer to the syndrome more and more as andropause and less and less as male menopause.

The incidence of mild cases of andropause approaches 95 percent of all men, and severe cases, about 10 percent. Severity is usually based on the degree of disability or disruption in the life of an andropausal man and his family. Well over 50 percent of all men acknowledge some degree of unhappiness and lowered productivity during the andropausal years.

The terms *andropause* and *viropause* are synonymous and used interchangeably, but *andropause* is the more commonly used in both local parlance and the medical literature in Europe and the United States. *Viropause* was first coined in a popular magazine article that appeared in 1993. The word *viropause* has the prefix "vir-," which appears in the Latin word *virilis,* meaning masculine. In English, *virile* means having the nature, properties, or qualities of an adult male. The origin of *andropause* is Greek. The root "andr-" or "andro-" denotes a relationship to man or the male. For example, the word *androgen* refers to any substance that possesses masculinizing characteristics. The suffix "-pause" is from the Latin *pausa* and the Greek *pausis.* In English, a pause denotes temporary inaction, so *andropause* connotes a temporary state in which a man's masculinity is sluggish or out of use.

There is an understandable tendency to use "andropause" and "testosterone deficiency" interchangeably, as if they both refer to the same event and set of symptoms in a man's life. In actuality, these are quite distinct and essentially unrelated phenomena, two separate medical conditions. As discussed in previous chapters, testosterone deficiency is a physical abnormality—an insufficient amount of the male hormone to supply the needs of the male body. Testosterone is necessary for normal function of the nervous and muscular systems. It's needed to delay bone demineralization and to maintain sexuality and a feeling of well-being.

Testosterone deficiency and andropause are basically different conditions, even though some of their symptoms overlap. Whereas testosterone deficiency is a physical condition, andropause is a psychological one. It is possible, though uncommon, for a man to be troubled by both conditions simultaneously. As testosterone deficiency becomes more closely defined in the future, better information concerning its incidence will be available. The definition will include blood levels as well as mental and bodily effects of the deficiency. Future research findings should make it easier to discern testosterone deficiency from andropause.

Testosterone deficiency usually produces annoying symptoms that prompt a man to seek medical attention. Between 5 and 20 percent of males, all ages considered, could benefit from testosterone replacement therapy. By contrast, andropause appears to occur in 50 to 75 percent of the men in the United States. Most cases go unrecognized, undiagnosed, and untreated.

The Causes of Andropause

American men are indoctrinated during their formative years to set high goals for themselves regarding financial achievement, high social status, and the regard of family, friends, and the community. Attaining high goals has become defined as the antithesis of failure. As men mature, the concept becomes deeply ingrained.

As men approach their middle years, they realize they have already lived half their lives—time is running out. At this time in life, most men begin assessing their achievements in relation to goals they set for themselves and the perceived success of their peers. Few men reach a zenith, and there is always someone, somewhere, who is more successful. This realization can be painfully disappointing. Men start acknowledging that they have been deluded, which makes them unhappy. When men reflect long or intensely on their disappointment, the result can be andropause. If they receive additional criticism from others, the sense of failure increases and self-esteem drops.

In a world where the desire for possessions and stature is continuously stroked by advertising, it's easy for men to feel an ever-increasing inadequacy. The intensity of our culture's marketing techniques purposely makes almost everyone feel in a constant state of dissatisfaction. And the human tendency toward hedonism adds to the discontent men feel about their achievements.

Failure in economic areas detracts from a man's sense of masculinity. There remains the idea that men who are under-achievers are weak. The feeling of lessened power contributes to the onset and protraction of the andropause.

For many men, the earliest signs of mental and physical aging initiate andropause. Men like to think they are impervious to the emotional response women have when they detect aging changes in their appearance. However, most men dislike balding, the shifting location of body fat, and a less erect posture. Aging and the anticipation of death are big negatives in any person's life, and an increased awareness of these events, instigated by aging changes, is distressing.

In American society, youth and evidence of youthfulness are given a high value. Advertising, clothing styles, entertainment, the news, and lifestyle promotion all contribute to the value and importance placed on youth. It's no wonder that when men become aware of even slight aging changes in their bodies, they are prone to some level of despondence.

Much of the nation's industrial output is directed to the younger members of society: sports pickup trucks, boats, bicycles, motorcycles, clothes, food and beverages, movies, music and most other forms of entertainment, participatory and televised sports, travel, vacation activities, youthening exercises, cosmetics, and so on. Men in andropause may fight aging changes with hair-loss retardants, vitamins, other food supplements, and youthful clothing. The most common mental aging change that often precipitates andropause is defective memory. Forgetting names and the details of events is, for most people, nothing more than an inconvenience, but for some men in their middle years, forgetfulness represents a deterioration of the thought process. As their concern increases, the symptoms of andropause intensify.

When men become aware of the changes that accompany aging, their minds go through a predictable process. The first step in this process is denial, a refusal to believe it's happening to them. The next is anger; men become angry at the cruelty and unfairness of life. The final step is an adjustment to the changes and an acknowledgment that many happy years remain. Men who are unable to make this adjustment often slip into andropause.

It is not unusual for men in their forties or fifties to develop deep fears that induce the andropause complex of changed behavior and unhappiness. Fear of discontentment often occurs at retirement age as men see their older friends experiencing failed retirement. Others fear financial decline or a decrease in respect from family and friends. When a man has a hormonal disturbance that interferes with his sexual function, the resulting angst and feelings of depression can also cause an andropausal condition. This is a situation in which testosterone deficiency can indirectly produce the psychological condition of andropause. Both unfounded and realistic fears may have causal effects on the andropause syndrome.

Testosterone Deficiency and Andropause

To eliminate the confusion that exists between testosterone deficiency and andropause, the general characteristics, incidence, onset, symptoms, severity, duration, diagnosis, treatment, and prognosis for each of the two conditions are summarized in Table 7-1.

General Characteristics

Testosterone deficiency is a physical abnormality consisting of insufficient male hormone to supply the needs of a man's body. Testosterone is needed for the normal functioning of the nervous and muscular systems. It's also necessary to delay bone demineralization and to maintain a feeling of well-being and sexuality.

Andropause is basically a psychological condition. A man in andropause is dysphoric or unhappy. There is a change in his psyche. He is unhappy with himself and his future. He reacts to this unhappiness with behavioral changes that often complicate and disrupt his life. The lives of those about him—family, friends, and colleagues—are also thrown into turmoil.

Table 7-1. A comparison of testosterone deficiency and andropause

	Andropause	Testosterone Deficiency
Basic characteristic	Psychological	Physical
Age at onset	40–60	55
Nature of onset	Gradual	Very gradual
Duration	1–5 years	Lifetime
Organs involved	Brain	Testes
Organs affected	Cardiovascular, neurological, digestive, genitourinary	Muscles, bone, genitalia
Physical changes	Psychosomatic	Muscle weakness, demineralization of bones
Psychological changes	Dysphoria, anxiety	Apathy, reduced libido
Diagnosis	Rule out physical abnormalities	Blood tests
Treatment	Mental self-adjustments	Testosterone replacement
Adjunctive treatment	Healthy lifestyle	Counseling when needed
Prognosis	Good	Excellent with treatment
Long-term care	Only if needed	Monitoring by physician

Incidence

Almost no scientific research has been done to determine how common these two conditions are or how frequently they occur. No reliable data concerning the incidence of either testosterone deficiency or andropause are available, but it is tempting to speculate.

Onset

Testosterone deficiency gradually occurs over decades, with symptoms becoming severe in a man's sixties or seventies. In rare cases, a severe illness or disease may rapidly result in testosterone deficiency. An illness of this magnitude produces other, much more disabling abnormalities, however, and the effects of testosterone deficiency can go unnoticed by the patient and his family. Obviously severe injuries to the testes drops the testosterone level quickly. A vasectomy, however, does not alter the testosterone-producing capability of the gonads.

The onset of andropause is most common between the ages of forty and sixty, but most frequently it appears in the late fifties when a man realizes his life is more than half over. The onset of andropause is usually gradual, but the symptoms can appear abruptly when something occurs that threatens a man's sense of security or masculinity.

Symptoms

The man experiencing testosterone deficiency is aware of some physical changes and the secondary symptoms caused by these changes. Some of these physical changes may include muscle weakness and lower endurance, increase or decrease in weight associated with change in appetite, less body hair, and impairment of sexual function (which produces more troublesome psychological disturbances as well). Other secondary symptoms can be changes in sleep pattern, feelings of either anxiety or depression, and increased irritability.

The symptoms of andropause and testosterone deficiency are similar, but the overall pattern of these symptoms is quite different. The underlying mood of a man in andropause is that of dysphoria. There is a general unhappiness and discontentment that can include fear of future financial and health failings, fear of loss of social status, fear of losing the love of others, and fear of waning sexuality.

The andropausal man usually has a poor self-image. Some of the ego-supporting features of his life are gone. He has a distorted sense of what is important in life, and his priorities are jumbled. If he has physical symptoms, they are psychosomatic and secondary to the disturbance and his mental unrest.

Severity

Severe testosterone deficiency usually produces symptoms that are distressing enough to a man to prompt him to seek medical attention. Milder deficiencies, however, often go unrecognized and undiagnosed. The severity of the symptoms correlates fairly well with the blood level of testosterone. There is a problem in trying to determine the incidence of the condition as it relates to chronological age. Between 5 and 20 percent of males, all ages considered, would benefit by testosterone replacement therapy.

The severity of the andropausal symptoms need to be considered when making a diagnosis. Andropause appears to occur in 50 to 75 percent of the men in the United States. Most cases go unrecognized, undiagnosed, and untreated by the man, his family, and his physician.

Duration

Testosterone deficiency is almost always a chronic abnormality and will persist for the rest of a man's life. If there is a severe but brief physical illness that reduces testosterone output, this deficiency will be reversed with the general recovery. Testicular shrinkage and the decreased output of testosterone by the gonads, which result from the injudicial use of anabolic android drugs, are partially reversible when the use of these substances is discontinued. The degree of recovery is probably related to gonadal function before using these drugs, dosage used, how long they were used, which ones were used, and the man's general health. The effects of testosterone deficiency are reversible by the use of replacement therapy.

Andropause lasts from a few months to several years. Typically the man gradually recovers in two or three years. Recovery is faster if he recognizes and accepts the diagnosis soon after the onset and makes an honest attempt to help himself or seek professional help. Understanding and support from friends may also shorten the duration of andropause.

Diagnosis

Testosterone deficiency is diagnosed by physical examination and, most important, by laboratory tests. The physical exam and laboratory tests are absolutely essential in establishing the diagnosis. Without the test results, the physician can only make an educated guess, but not a diagnosis of testosterone deficiency. Milder deficiencies often go unrecognized and undiagnosed. Severity of symptoms correlates fairly well with the blood level of testosterone.

Andropause cannot be diagnosed by a physical examination or laboratory tests, although these are helpful to rule out physical conditions that imitate andropause, such as hormonal imbalances (including testosterone deficiency), heart disease, dietary deficiencies, and muscular disorders. The diagnosis is based on the patient's history, that is, what the man tells his physician. This includes his description of how he feels, changes in his behavior, and how it is affecting others. The history usually includes secondary symptoms of a physical nature referred to as psychosomatic conditions.

Treatment

Treatment of testosterone deficiency is more direct and dependable. Once there is laboratory evidence of the condition, treatment can begin without delay. The treatment includes the education of the patient as well as the replacement of testosterone by one or more methods of administration. Because the man and other members of his family can have an emotional response to the illness, some psychotherapy may be in order for a short time.

As in many conditions, the best treatment for andropause is the elimination of the cause. Since the causes are of a psychological nature, the treatment should be directed to easing the anxiety, dysphoria, fears, and reduced self-esteem. The andropausal man must make an in-depth inventory of his strengths, weaknesses, and fears and then deal with them realistically. If he is experiencing sexual deterioration, professional help is needed. If there is a physical reason for this dysfunction, a diagnosis and appropriate treatment should be used. Not commonly but occasionally, the physical abnormality may actually be a testosterone deficiency. If physical causes for sexual problems are ruled out, then the psychological approach is in order.

Prognosis

Response to replacement therapy for testosterone deficiency is almost always satisfactory. A few months may pass until the correct dose of testosterone and most acceptable route of administration are determined. Over the years dosage adjustments may require reassessment. Regular physical examinations and laboratory testing must be performed to make certain no serious side effects are developing during therapy. This evaluation is usually part of the routine annual health inventory and examination.

With appropriate management, most men can expect a complete recovery from andropause. The management may consist of their own efforts, help from friends and/or family, and, if these are not adequate, professional assistance.

Many medical conditions are subject to relapses of mild to moderate severity, and andropause is no exception. When a relapse does occur, the treatment is essentially the same as for the primary episode, though it is of less intensity and requires a shorter period of therapy. As with other abnormalities, both physical and psychological, if the underlying causes persist (e.g., unresolved marital conflict, fears and worries, sexual inadequacies), the illness may become chronic.

CHAPTER EIGHT

Beyond Hormones

Understanding
Sexual Dysfunction in Men

- **Premature Ejaculation**
- **Libido**
- **Orgasmic Failure**
- **Impotence**
- **Treatment for Impotence**

- **Drugs and Sexual Dysfunction**
- **Prostate Disease and Sexuality**

F ew men suffering with sexual problems seek help from their doctors. Probably less than 5 percent of male patients in urologists' and primary physicians' offices give sexual dysfunction as their chief complaint. Most cases of sexual dysfunction are detected when a doctor asks during a general physical exam, "Do you have any sexual problems?" Men seldom volunteer this information unless asked directly about it.

Women are much more likely to acknowledge their sexual problems than men, but their problems often result from their partners' performance. These same male partners will deny any sexual dysfunction.

Premature Ejaculation

The only common sexual problem usually reported by young and middle-aged men is premature ejaculation. Erection failure is the most common complaint of older men, though some may experience premature ejaculation also. Men generally don't consider this a problem for themselves, but about half of them express concern about "going off before my partner has come."

The use of local anesthetic cream applied to the penis to reduce sensitivity has been used but found to be of limited value. Though not approved for this purpose by the FDA, antidepressant drugs such as Prozac have been found effective in the treatment of premature ejaculation. One of the side effects of these medications is a delay of orgasm and, occasionally, no orgasm, even with prolonged thrusting. By natural evolution, clinicians started prescribing antidepressants for premature ejaculation.

Libido

Low Libido

If a man is not sexually attracted to his partner physically and emotionally, no tests, medications, or counseling are going to be successful in producing a healthy libido. Androgens can increase libido, but both the patient and the physician should realize that this is not a substitute for a libido that develops out of the feelings of love and affection. If lack of attraction is the problem and the man increases his libido with testosterone replacement therapy, it may create a new problem. The man may seek sexual gratification with someone other than his committed partner.

It cannot be assumed that low testosterone levels are responsible for low libido. Poor overall physical and mental health often decrease the libido. Many chronic illnesses lower libido, as do stress and anxiety. A common symptom of depression in both men and women is a decrease in libido. It is not unusual for a depression patient to report absolutely no interest in sex whatsoever. Various over-the-counter and prescription drugs may also lower libido.

High Libido

There is great variation in the normal range of libidos. Contrary to popular opinion, an overabundance of testosterone does not result in an abnormally high libido. No known conditions produce excessive amounts of testosterone, and no abnormalities of the testis cause excessive hormone production. Abnormal sexual behavior is also not caused by an excessive amount of testosterone. Too much testosterone would result in the same undesirable side effects as excessive anabolic steroid ingestion: abnormally aggressive behavior, liver and other organ disease, and increased risk for cardiovascular problems. It would not, however, result in a man becoming excessively libidinous.

There has never been any need to develop a treatment for excessive testosterone in men. Some forensic medicine specialists, however, are interested in using antitestosterone drugs to lower libido to help in the management of criminals guilty of sexual crime. Sexual crimes are usually caused by mental disturbances, not physical or sexual problems, but reducing or eliminating libido in men who commit such crimes, regardless of their normal libido level, is of some use.

Differing Libido Levels in Couples

Libido is an extremely important element of sexuality. The correspondence of the libido levels of the partners in a physical relationship has considerable influence on that relationship. Some incongruity is normal, but a wide disparity can contribute significantly to a breakdown in the relationship. On the other hand, if the libido levels of the two are similar, the relationship can withstand a considerable amount of other pressure without collapsing. Fortunately, a significant difference is usually correctable if both partners are willing. Less common and more difficult to treat is the woman's need and desire for more sexual activity when her partner "just can't do it like he used to." Almost always women will express sympathy and claim, "We still have a good love and are very close to each other."

The older man's most common sexual complaint is impotence. If both he and his partner have low libidos, nothing needs to be done. But if his partner has a high libido, some form of medical or psychological intervention may be appropriate.

When there is a troubling disparity in libido that's not helped by conversation and agreement, then outside help is in order. If one member of a couple wants sex somewhat more than the other, usually an agreement to follow a middle road—

both giving a little—is an adequate compromise. However, if the disparity is great, outside professional help, from a counselor or a physician, should be sought.

Hormonal therapy can be an effective treatment for disparate libido levels. An understanding and knowledgeable physician may prescribe testosterone for a woman or a man with a low libido. This approach is used fairly often when there is a libido disparity in young couples but is not considered as often for older couples, although there's no reason for it not to be. Before medical therapy is prescribed, there must be a reasonable certainty that the low libido isn't the result of some other factor such as a partner's poor hygiene or an absence of love.

Besides the testosterone decrease, other causes of dropping libido as men age are possible. General health status is the most important of these. A man who is debilitated even slightly has a decreased libido. ("Dirty old men" are usually pretty healthy.) Slowed flow of oxygenated blood to nerve cells, especially the brain, no doubt, decreases libido. Reduced response to erotic stimuli plays a role in this change. Fortunately, for older couples who have a good relationship, the sexual expression of love becomes less important. The answer to the relational problems of older couples is the same as for young couples—communication.

Orgasmic Failure

A tremendous crescendo of physical and mental activity occurs during sexual excitement. The sensation is enjoyable, but if not terminated in a satisfactory orgasm, the mental tension is unrelieved. Men have difficulty putting this into words, but anyone who has experienced interrupted or failed orgasms is familiar with it and strongly desires to avoid a recurrence. The anxiety and tension subside way too slowly.

The inability to reach an orgasm after prolonged thrusting is very frustrating to men and often a source of considerable anxiety, especially if it occurs frequently. The problem often perpetuates itself. If a man has had a recent orgasmic failure, on his next sexual encounter he will be more occupied with fear of sexual failure than with love and affection. His erotic thoughts will be displaced by worry.

Like erections, having a vigorous orgasm is a symbol of masculinity to a man. In most men, the first or second erectile or orgasmic failure is enough to introduce an element of fear: fear that the condition may be progressing and fear that the failure signals the beginning of an asexual existence.

Getting treatment for fear of sexual failure is as important as getting treatment for a physical sexual disorder. The man needs to understand the cause of the failure and receive reassurance. An injection of testosterone can be an effective part of the support system. Its libido-enhancing effect allows the man to enter into the next encounter with vigor and self-assurance, allowing the mental block to be removed. Testosterone does not cure orgasmic failure, but it can boost a man's self-esteem and confidence, which help him overcome any psychological causes for the failure.

Most clinicians and researchers believe orgasmic dysfunction results from an abnormality in the thought process. This may explain why so little is known about treating orgasm dysfunction, since psychological research has always lagged behind physical research.

Evidence that orgasm is a psychological function is found in how psychogenic medicines affect orgasm. Sedatives, especially the barbiturates, delay or prevent orgasms. Excessive alcohol, which is a nervous system depressant, interferes with orgasm as well as erection. Antidepressant drugs delay or prevent orgasms in up to 30 percent of men, which suggests that the neurochemical serotonin plays some role in bringing about an orgasm.

Fortunately, orgasm dysfunction is not common—fortunate because knowledge about its treatment is so limited. Sufficient research has been done regarding the physical events during orgasm—which muscles contract, how ejaculation occurs, and what happens to blood pressure, pulse rate, and respirations just before and during orgasm—but we know very little about the mental events involved. Some of the thoughts that promote orgasm are love, affection, awareness of exciting sensory stimuli, and any form of eroticism. Orgasm requires intensely focused thinking (even more intensely focused thoughts than are required for erection).

Mental interruptions can disrupt a man's ability to have an orgasm. Absence of love and affection can interfere, but less in men than in women. Fears of various sorts can interfere. In addition to the fear of failure, other fears include interruption by others in the household (including children entering the room), overexertion leading to a heart attack, undesired impregnation of the woman, and inability to bring the partner to orgasm before the man ejaculates. These are the same fears as those responsible for erectile dysfunction.

Fatigue, especially mental fatigue, delays or prevents orgasms. Most men who only occasionally experience orgasm failure usually relate it to tiredness. Orgasm failures are infrequent in the morning hours or when the couple is on vacation.

Impotence

If we can believe the media and anecdotal reports, the number of men suffering from impotence is larger than previously believed. It has been estimated that twenty-five million American men suffer occasional impotence. Of men surveyed by Kinsey, almost 7 percent between ages forty-five and fifty-five reported impotence, and one of four men is impotent by the age of seventy-five.

The word *impotence* generally indicates an inability to copulate, but in medical terms it means the inability to achieve or maintain a penile erection of sufficient quality to engage in successful sexual intercourse. There is nothing more distressing to a man than being unable to develop an erection when he and his partner are ready for sexual intercourse.

The exact relationship between testosterone and impotence is not well understood, not because of inadequate research but because the problem is extremely complex. To begin such a study, the researcher is immediately forced to accept the widely recognized fact that there is more than one cause of impotence.

Psychological distress is the most common cause of impotence as well as orgasmic failure. There are also a number of nonhormonal, physical causes for impotence such as diabetes, nerve diseases, blood vessel diseases, abnormalities of the arteries in the penis, and general debility. Diabetes mellitus is a notorious cause of impotence. Diabetes, unless there are complications, usually gives no warning symptoms. Uncontrolled diabetes is a common cause of neuritis, an inflammation of the nerves, and the resulting nerve damage is a recognized cause of impotence.

The arteries in men with uncontrolled diabetes age at a rapid rate. Uncontrolled diabetes is a frequent cause of either partial or complete artery obstruction (atherosclerosis), including the arteries to the penis. When diabetes is under tight control, the arteries age at approximately the same rate as those of the nondiabetic person. No medications are effective in expanding the internal dimensions of arteries obstructed by atherosclerosis, so this condition is treatable only by surgery. Early diagnosis and control of diabetes are essential to preventing impotence from artery-related abnormalities.

Cigarette smoking damages arteries throughout the body. In skin it increases wrinkling, in the heart it contributes to the blockage of the coronary arteries, and in the penis it impairs the function of the arteries of erection. High lipid levels (cholesterol) similarly contribute to artery disease.

The use of tobacco has both a short- and long-term detrimental effect on erectile function. Its long-term effect on arteries has been recognized and reported by many researchers. A report in 1988 showing the short-term effects stated that smoking two cigarettes before testing prevented the induction of an erection and reduced the pressures within the distensible tissue of the penis following penile injections of papaverine (a commonly used drug to produce erections). Men who have any impotence should avoid cigarette smoking for a period of time before engaging in sexual activity.

Many medications, both over-the-counter and prescription, also interfere with erectile function. These include some of the medications for high blood pressure, indigestion, allergies, colds, depression, and anxiety. Both legal and illegal drugs are common antagonists of satisfactory erectile performance. Acute intoxication and chronic drug use are well-known detractors of good erections.

Impotence is a symptom, not a diagnosis. To make a diagnosis requires medical investigation including a medical history, physical examination, blood tests, and possibly imaging studies. An exact diagnosis must be established to treat the condition successfully.

Impotence due to impaired blood flow requires treating the arteries; impotence due to hypothyroidism responds to thyroid replacement; impotence caused by the blocking effect of a medication needs adjustment of the mediation regimen; impotence resulting from depression needs antidepression medication or psychological counseling; impotence from other emotional causes needs targeted therapy.

Treatment for Impotence

Only about 10 percent of the two million men suffering with impotence seek treatment. Testosterone replacement therapy is one of the treatments of choice for cases with a psychological cause because it increases libido, elevates mood, and improves a man's self-perceived masculinity.

Testosterone

Testosterone has been oversold as a treatment for impotence. The effect of androgens on libido and sexual behavior has been well established, but their effect on erectile functions is less clear. There are probably many cases of impotence in which testosterone deficiency has some role but few cases where it's the sole cause of the defect. In the lay literature, testosterone is promoted for impotence, but the medical literature is much less optimistic.

Dating back to the early decades of this century, there are many anecdotal reports on the wonders of testosterone for curing impotence. It is no wonder many men seek hormonal treatment to increase their potency and restore their manhood. Unfortunately, some physicians are willing to supply the treatment without good clinical evidence of a testosterone deficiency. In addition, charlatans and black marketers make testosterone available without a prescription.

The anecdotal reports suggesting testosterone cures impotence don't stand up to scientific scrutiny. It is nearly impossible to eliminate the placebo effect in these reports, but physicians still have good reason to use testosterone to treat many cases of impotence. The well-documented increase in libido is indirectly but definitely a factor in keeping erectile function. Libido doesn't just mean an increase in desire for sexual activity but also a greater enthusiasm for the act of coitus itself. The man enjoys greater vigor, both mentally and physically, and more intensity. Improvement in these factors can be effective in eliminating the psychological element of impotence.

The muscle change and feeling of well-being from testosterone also come into play. Testosterone replacement increases muscle mass and strength. Most men relate muscle size and strength to masculinity. Testosterone improves self-esteem by changing weakness to strength, feelings of inadequacy to assurance, and gloom of sexual failure to euphoria of sexual prowess. The improvement helps counteract psychogenic impotence. Elevated self-esteem promotes happiness, assertiveness, and productivity; increases energy; lessens fatigue; and produces a greater appreciation for all good things. Regardless of other causes of impotence, a high level of testosterone contributes positively to some degree in managing the condition.

The benefits of testosterone therapy for erectile dysfunction occur gradually over a period of a few months, although some patients report almost immediate improvement in their penile function. This early response is usually attributed to the placebo effect and suggests the presence of a psychological factor in addition to the testosterone deficiency. The improvement in libido occurs soon after starting replacement therapy so it appears that improved libido indirectly improves erectile function.

Other Drugs

As one might expect, there is tremendous interest by patients and pharmaceutical manufacturers in drugs that improve sexual function. Some agents taken orally have received some recognition.

Yohimbine is an alkaloid from plant sources suggested to work on a certain part of the brain where there are a number of neurotransmitters that act to regulate erections. It has been in use for more than a hundred years but only recently has been subject to scientific investigation. When yohimbine was tested on men with psychogenic impotence, 62 percent had positive results as compared with 16 percent using a placebo. The reports have stimulated research into the same general class of drugs as Viagra (sildenafil). Adding Trazadone (originally introduced as an antidepressant, but known to be a serotonin antagonist) to yohimbine has been tried with some success, but this approach has not yet been reported in the medical literature.

Researchers have also shown interest in the role dopamine plays in sexual function. Dopamine, naturally manufactured in the body, acts as a neurotransmitter in the brain. Some drugs tested to facilitate the function of dopamine for improving erections are L-Dopa, Deprenyl, Apomorphine, Pergolide, and Fenfluramine.

Nitroglycerin has been used for decades to improve cardiovascular function to relieve angina (chest pain). For years it was administered by holding a dissolvable tablet under the tongue. More recently, when a prolonged effect is desired, skin application is used in the form of a skin patch or a paste. There is now interest in using nitroglycerin to induce erections of the penis. Pastes containing nitroglycerin or related compounds have been applied to the base of the penis with some favorable results in treating impotence. Topical glyceryltrinitrate causes measurable penile arterial dilation in impotent men. If this topical approach proves effective, it will probably be used primarily for impotence of vascular causes, especially if blood flow obstruction is partial and not more advanced.

A new, noninjectable, and painless drug delivery system for alprostadil, a synthetic form of the hormone prostaglandin E, has just been approved by the FDA. Alprostadil relaxes the smooth muscles in the penis, which allows blood to flow in and cause an erection. Both safe and effective, this new method involves inserting a tiny drug-carrying pellet into the urethra. A slender plunger carrying the pellet is pushed an inch and a half into the end of the penis. Sixty-five percent of the impotent men ages twenty-seven to eighty-eight using the plunger in test trials were able to get an hour-long erection, typically within five minutes. Only 11 percent of the testers had the side effect of a dull ache in their penis, which was caused by the medicine, not the insertion.

Nondrug Treatments

A number of other medical options are available for treating impotence. The six treatments that have been approved and are available by prescription are inflatable implants, bendable rods, insertable pellets, vacuum pumps, penile injections, and prosthetic implants. A vacuum device or an injection of a medication (papaverine) into the penis will create an erection, although it will not correct the underlying abnormality. Some causes, however, are not correctable, and the best that can be done is the use of symptomatic treatment. For example, impotence due to severe artery obstruction to the penis can be treated with a penile implant.

Although the various methods all have a good success rate, 80 to 95 percent, they all have drawbacks also. While injections into the penis act quickly, usually producing an erection in three to five minutes, some of them cause a dull pain. There have also been reports of liver problems, cardiovascular difficulties, penile fibrosis (tough fibrous tissue accumulating in the penis), and priapism (sustained, unwanted erection) from the injections. One fairly new injectable treatment, Caverject from Upjohn, has an 80 percent success rate. In spite of the improved convenience, there is still a 40 percent dropout rate because so many men don't like to inject themselves in the penis. It also is costly at up to $25 a shot. The inflatable implants are cumbersome and can fail and cause infection. The vacuum pumps cost up to $400, and, even though they have a 95 percent success rate, only 5 to 10 percent of impotent men choose them. There's a 25 percent dropout rate among users. A prosthetic penile implant requires a $15,000 operation, and the silicone in the implant may be hazardous.

The corpus cavernosum (the distensible spongy tissue) of the penis has specialized muscles that keep the penis from filling with blood. Erection occurs when the muscles are relaxed. During sexual stimulation, nitric oxide is released, which initiates a two-stage chemical reaction that allows relaxation of these muscles. Nitric oxide (not to be confused with nitrous oxide, used as an anesthetic by dentists) is produced by the nerve endings that go to the blood supply and by the spongy tissue of the penis. It is a potent poison but only lasts three seconds after it is produced. It paralyzes and relaxes the muscles of the blood vessels in the penis so they can expand in width, allowing the 600 percent increase in blood flow that occurs in the erection process. Men with physical impotence from causes like diabetes and strokes do not produce sufficient nitric oxide to produce an erection, but nitric oxide can't be administered directly because of its poisonous nature.

Most of the injectable medications for impotence, like prostaglandin E-1 and papaverine with Regitine, work by stimulating the production of nitric oxide. In contrast, the oral medication sildenafil works directly on the muscles.

The Food and Drug Administration (FDA) approved the use of a noninvasive treatment for impotence in late 1996, and it became available by prescription in January 1997. The product has been named MUSE (medicated urethral system for erection) and contains Alprostadil, which is one of the ingredients used for injection into the penis to produce an erection. The onset of erections is within five to ten minutes after insertion, and the duration is approximately thirty to sixty minutes. The recommended maximum frequency of use is twice within twenty-four hours.

MUSE consists of a medicated pellet for placement in the urethra of the penis. The applicator is a small tube that is inserted into the urethra. At the end is a medicated pellet that is released into the penis by thumb pressure on a protruding button. The applicator is then withdrawn and discarded. The pellet is available in four strengths: 125, 250, 500, and 1,000 micrograms. The effective dose varies from patient to patient and is determined by trial and error in consultation with a physician.

For best results, the man should not lie down for ten minutes after insertion. This sitting or standing period of time may be incorporated into foreplay. After this initial ten minutes, any position may be assumed with no interference in effectiveness of the system. If a man wishes to terminate an erection, he can apply ice packs to his inner thighs.

The adverse effects caused by the injection of Alprostadil—pain and bruising—are avoided by using the urethral route of administration. The side effects of MUSE are discomfort, usually mild and transient, and slight bleeding. In the research studies, 7 percent of the patients discontinued using the system because of the side effects, as compared with 37 percent using the injection route. MUSE has no contraceptive effect, nor does it impede the transmission of disease. Less than 6 percent of the men's female partners in one study reported burning or itching, but this reaction could be due to the increased frequency of coitus when MUSE is used.

Drugs and Sexual Dysfunction

Abnormal sexual function occurs as a side effect with a large number of drugs and medications. The abnormalities are caused by drugs working on the nervous system, the vascular system, and hormone production. See Chapter 13, including Figure 13-1, for a detailed discussion of drugs' effects on sexual function.

Prostate Disease and Sexuality

The prostate gland is a solid structure that surrounds the urethra located at the base of the urinary bladder in men. The healthy adult prostate is the size and shape of a walnut. The role played by the prostate in sexual intercourse is relatively minor. It supplies, and secretes into the urethra, a lubricant for intercourse. This lubricating fluid also carries the sperm during ejaculation. Sexuality does not affect the prostate in any way, but prostate disease, more specifically, the treatment of prostate disease, can cause sexual problems.

There are three common prostate disorders: inflammation, benign growth, and cancer. Prostate inflammation, known as *prostatitis,* is often caused by bacterial infection. In almost all cases, the bacteria involved are those that normally inhabit the human intestine, the most common of which is *E. coli.* The mechanism by which bacteria invade the prostate is not conclusively understood.

Another type of prostatitis, referred to as *nonbacterial prostatitis,* is eight times more common than the bacterial condition. The symptoms of both are the same: low backache, pelvic pain, and discomfort in the area between the scrotum and anus. The cause of nonbacterial prostatitis has also not been conclusively identified.

Having prostatitis does not increase a man's chance of having benign prostate enlargement (hyperplasia) or prostate cancer, and prostatitis does not affect sexuality or performance. Treating prostatitis, with or without antibiotics, does not impact sexuality in any way.

Sexual habits have never been incriminated as a cause of prostatitis, but regular ejaculation has been suggested as a way to reduce recurrent infections of the prostate. During ejaculation, the fluid from the prostate flows into the urethra and composes part of the ejected semen. It's suspected that more frequent emptying of the prostate decreases the bacterial concentration in the gland.

Benign prostatic hyperplasia (BPH) is a common disorder of the prostate. *Hyperplasia* refers to an abnormal increase in the number of cells. BPH is present in 50 percent of sixty-year-old men and 90 percent of those reaching eighty-five. It causes symptoms of the urinary bladder, most often that of getting up at night to urinate. Other symptoms include hesitancy in starting urination and decreased force in the urinary stream. Dribbling afterward can also be an extremely annoying symptom.

BPH is not caused by sexual activity, nor does abstinence or infrequency of coitus have any influence on the condition. BPH does not increase the likelihood of the development of prostate cancer. There are both medical and surgical treatments that are used to decrease the symptoms. The drug Proscar (finosteride) reduces the size of the prostate by 20 to 25 percent after three to six months of use. There is a small side effect: it decreases libido in approximately 5 to 10 percent of patients.

A group of medications called alpha antagonists has been approved by the FDA for treating BPH, though originally they were used to treat high blood pressure. Reportedly 70 percent effective, they work by reducing the tone of certain muscles that have an obstructing effect on the flow of urine through the prostate and the bladder neck. Side effects are uncommon. A few may experience dizziness on the higher doses, but less than 1 percent have any sexual dysfunction.

Surgical treatment for BPH is known as *prostatectomy*, and it often results in retrograde ejaculation. In this condition, the semen flows backward and travels up into the bladder during ejaculation. The semen is then expelled with urination. Some men find this disturbing, but most men are unaware of any change in the sensations of orgasm. Some men and their sexual partners find this a convenience—there is less need to wipe away the fluids following coitus.

The occasional patient experiences impotence following surgery for BPH, and some researchers attribute it to psychogenic factors. Most studies have found that patients with postoperative impotence had underlying erectile dysfunction before their procedure. Older men are more likely to have complications from the surgery, according to published data. Surgery performed through the urethra, known as transurethral resection prostatectomy (TURP), is much less likely to result in impotence than other approaches to prostatectomy.

Carcinoma, or cancer, of the prostate is rare before age fifty, but the incidence subsequently increases with age. It is the most common malignancy of men in the United States (other than skin cancers) and the second most common cause of cancer death in men. The etiology is unknown. There has never been any risk relationship to sexual practices or habits. Frequent sexual activity neither increases nor decreases the risk of developing prostate cancer.

In recent years, the widespread use of a test to screen levels of prostate-specific antigen (PSA) has increased the awareness of both the public and the medical profession to the subject of prostate cancer. PSA is produced by certain cells of the prostate, and it normally liquefies the semen. More is produced when BPH, infection, or cancer are present. Cancer produces ten times as much PSA as BPH.

Medical researchers and clinicians are in disaccord about the use of PSA testing for various reasons. One problem is the high incidence of false positives and false negatives with the test. There is no agreement about who should have the screening blood test, what age the screening should begin, what additional studies should be performed if the test is positive, or even what constitutes a positive report. Most physicians use the test judiciously along with the digital rectal examination in advising patients and selecting management.

The choice of prostate cancer management and treatment depends on a number of factors, such as the patient's age and general health, the type of cancer, and the extent of the malignancy. Treatment of prostate cancer often does affect a man's sexuality.

Considerable psychological trauma ensues when a man first learns he has any sort of malignancy. That reaction, by itself, affects his sexuality. If the malignancy is prostate cancer, he very soon wonders how the disease and treatment will affect his sexuality. Some men take the bad news in stride and experience no change in their sexuality. At the other end of the spectrum, some men may have a total loss of libido and/or become impotent from the moment they hear the bad news due to the psychological trauma. The response of most men falls somewhere in between, and their sexuality, from a psychological standpoint, oscillates from day to day.

CHAPTER NINE

Pumping Up Chemically

Synthetic Steroids and Their Relationship to Masculine Characteristics

- **Anabolic Steroids**
- **Anabolic Steroid Use by Athletes**
- **The Harmful Effects of Anabolic Steroid Use**
- **Overdosing on Steroids**
- **Safe Alternatives to Anabolic Steroids**

A n old magazine advertisement pictured, in the first frame, a bully kicking beach sand on a pretty girl while her skinny boyfriend watches with obvious frustration. The boyfriend then uses the Charles Atlas weight training program to enlarge his muscles. In the last frame, the boyfriend, now with bulging muscles, scares off the bully to win the pretty girl's heart.

Advertising today uses a similar technique to sell weight training courses as well as exercise apparatuses, weight loss plans, and nutritional supplements. Just about every cable station carries an ad for a mail-order abdominal muscle builder. These muscle-oriented ads insinuate that large muscles are evidence not only of strength but also of virility, power, sexual prowess, youth, and even greater economic potential.

Early muscle ads were all directed at men, but in recent times, women have also been caught up by the concept. The ads tell them that larger, more defined muscles are physically more attractive, especially to men, and indicate good health. Some women are encouraged in their muscle-building efforts by muscular male acquaintances.

People are impatient by nature and don't appreciate delayed gratification. They want what they want *now*. The impatient desire for muscles of superior size and strength induces some to use anabolic steroids to achieve their goal more quickly.

Anabolic Steroids

Steroid is a generic term that is often misused. Steroids are a large group of naturally occurring organic compounds that includes cholesterol, bile products, adrenal hormones, and sex hormones. There are numerous types of steroids such as anabolic steroids, sex steroids, and adrenal steroids. Cortisone and its many derivatives are adrenal steroids.

The anabolic steroids are synthetic male sex hormones derived from, and chemically similar to, testosterone. Both have similar effects on the body. *Anabolic* means that the steroid has the characteristic of increasing constructive metabolism, such as building new muscle tissue. Although testosterone and the anabolic steroids are both hormones, testosterone is a natural substance synthesized from cholesterol, while anabolic steroids are synthetically produced chemicals.

All steroids, including cortisone products, increase the appetite. Part of the anabolic effect is an increase in the metabolism in some of the body tissues. Increased metabolism increases the body's demand for food (calories).

Testosterone is a naturally occurring anabolic steroid and was the first chemical used as an externally administered anabolic agent. For various reasons, mostly related to side effects, it was never a practical choice in medical treatment. A few dozen years ago, laboratories of pharmaceutical companies began experimenting with related chemicals. The hope was to develop drugs that would have an anabolic effect but without the androgenic results. In synthesizing anabolic steroids, the chemists' goal has been to retain the muscle-building characteristics of testosterone but without the masculinizing and psychological effects. Their success has been limited. (See the Appendix for a further discussion of anabolic steroids.)

Anabolic Steroid Use by Athletes

Since the early 1950s, athletes have also used anabolic steroids in the hope of enhancing performance despite efforts to discourage or ban the practice. A study of testosterone and the brain demonstrated that the psychological stress associated with athletic competition stimulates a natural increase in the amount of circulating testosterone, especially for older athletes. The underlying mechanism of muscle enlargement by weight training involves slightly injuring the muscles. The recovery process results in bigger and stronger muscles. The recovery takes two to three days, so lifters do their exercises at intervals of three days or more. Though never scientifically proven, a belief persists that anabolic steroids facilitate this injury/recovery/growth process. The effect of anabolic steroids is expressed in the nitrogen balance in the muscle tissue. A positive nitrogen balance benefits muscle building, and a negative nitrogen balance detracts.

Since steroids provide a synthetic strength and endurance advantage, many sports competitions, such as the Olympics, test athletes for steroid use before they are allowed to compete. Evidence of unusual quantities of any of the androgens in the bloodstream, testosterone or anabolic steroids, will disqualify an athlete from competition. The most widely used drug test, and the one accepted by the International Olympic Committee, is a urinalysis test that looks at the ratio between testosterone and a substance called epitestosterone, which is a byproduct of testosterone produced by the body. A ratio of greater than 6 constitutes an offense.

It has been discovered, however, that some environmental factors can bias the test so that it may appear an athlete is using drugs when he or she is not. For example, anabolic-androgenic steroids are commonly used as growth promoters in livestock, so athletes who consume meat containing such hormone residues may risk failing a sports drug test. In clinical studies, 50 percent of subjects tested positive (a ratio above 6) twenty-four hours after eating meat from hormone-treated chickens. Eating meat containing small amounts of injected hormone may constitute a serious liability for athletes. A more reliable test, which evaluates the urinary ratio between testosterone and a substance called 17 alpha-hydroxyprogesterone, is under investigation as an alternate test.

The Harmful Effects of Anabolic Steroid Use

The injudicious use of anabolic steroids can be harmful to both body and mind. In 1993, more than one million users or former users of anabolic steroids were estimated in the United States. All anabolic steroids have often unwelcome, androgenic (masculinizing) effects if given in sufficient doses and over a prolonged period of time. The apparently reversible short-term side effects include acne, hair loss, reduced libido, increased irritability, and masculinization in women. Prolonged use of anabolic steroids might lead to harmful effects on the heart, brain, eyes, kidneys, and skin. When oral steroid preparations are taken, the liver is often affected. Both anabolic steroids and testosterone are known to adversely affect the liver when taken orally, especially in larger doses, but liver disease is much more common in users of anabolic steroids than in testosterone users because the anabolic steroids are usually taken orally and in huge doses.

Excessive testosterone doses could have some of the same unfavorable side effects as anabolic steroids, but because of the way testosterone is administered, it's almost impossible to take a dangerous dose. Orally administered testosterone and the related synthetic steroid compounds move directly to the liver via the bloodstream, which means they arrive in the liver in an unaltered state. Androgens are metabolized (processed) in the liver and affect this organ in various ways. Liver cysts have been extensively reported. Liver tumors and inflammation are less commonly reported, but these conditions are potentially very serious. Liver changes similar to those in alcoholics can have devastating effects. When the liver becomes diseased, some of the blood on the way to the heart is rerouted to vessels in the esophagus. These vessels dilate and are subject to rupture, causing hemorrhaging.

Body builders report increased libido while on anabolic steroids. This is not surprising considering that therapeutic doses of testosterone are used for treatment of gonadal insufficiency, but impotence has also been reported when men are on large doses of steroids.

The hormonal effects of the anabolic steroids have been extensively reported in the medical literature. Anabolic steroids suppress the normal production and utilization of sex hormones in men's bodies. The androgen levels fall when steroids are being used because the level of gonadotropic (gonad-stimulating) hormone, which is responsible for stimulating the production of male sex hormones, falls. Thyroid gland function becomes impaired, testosterone production is reduced, and the testes shrink. Extremely small gonads have been found in men on large sustained doses of anabolic steroids. Sterility is a common complication.

Many instances of ruptured tendons, ligaments, and muscles occur in steroid users. Although this is not unusual in body builders and athletes who are putting strain on their muscles and joints, these tissues may be at greater risk with excessive doses of anabolic steroids.

Significant unfavorable changes in the lipid levels occur with anabolic steroid use. The HDL ("good" cholesterol) is lowered, while the LDL ("bad" cholesterol) is elevated. These changes have undesirable effects on the arteries.

The cardiovascular consequences of android steroids are widely recognized. The heart muscle changes in ways that can contribute to heart disease and even death. Steroid overuse induces an unfavorable enlargement and thickening of the left ventricle of the heart. A paralyzing stroke was reported in a thirty-four-year-old man who was using steroids for four years. This condition may have occurred because androgens increase the bone marrow's production of red blood cells, which may be a factor in the formation of thromboses (clots).

Psychological changes are also common and widely recognized in regular, large-dose users of anabolic steroids. The aggressive nature of anabolic steroid users is probably an extension of the feeling of well-being that comes with smaller doses of testosterone. The mild euphoria created by correct doses of testosterone can be exaggerated by overdosing with the anabolic steroids to the point of unnaturally aggressive behavior. Testosterone and its derivatives do increase aggression. Even though increased aggressiveness might be desirable on the playing field, it can be disruptive in the home and personal relationships. Body builders on steroids, and their families, are familiar with fits of anger. Commonly called "roid rages" by the wives and girlfriends of steroid-using body builders, these episodes have sometimes resulted in physical attacks on women.

Psychological studies suggest that certain personality characteristics increase the potential of anabolic steroid abuse in some men. Several articles describe narcissistic personality traits. Other characteristics are perfectionism, ineffectiveness, and low self-esteem. Suicides of athletes and patients who have been using anabolic steroids have also been reported.

Anabolic steroids are not typically used by younger teenagers, but if children use them before they reach full stature, they will not grow to their full height. Steroids close the bone epiphyses, the parts of bones from which growth occurs, so steroids prevent normal growth.

Some medical literature characterizes the use of anabolic steroids as an addiction. The federal Drug Enforcement

Agency (DEA) classifies anabolic steroids as Class III drugs. This is the same class that contains codeine, sedatives, and tranquilizers, most of which are addictive. It is true that suddenly stopping anabolic steroids does result in withdrawal symptoms. Steroids produce a reverse negative calcium and nitrogen balance that stimulates feelings of well-being and increased appetite. It is understandable, psychologically as well as physically, that a man whose big muscles and mild euphoria disappear with the cessation of steroids would be in distress.

With a suitable diet and present-day medications, both the short-term effects and damage from long-term steroid use are thought to be reversible in most cases. After a suitable period of abstinence, the liver damage, the cardiovascular effects, the hormonal changes, and the personality disruption disappear. The depression that occurs following the withdrawal of anabolic steroids can successfully be treated with an antidepressant such as Prozac.

The excessive use of anabolic steroids is of concern to the nation's health because there is no information about their long-term effects, even after steroids are discontinued, whereas the long-term effects of testosterone are well known and understood. Human use of testosterone has been studied for a century, but the use of anabolic steroid studies didn't begin until the last two or three decades.

Overdosing on Steroids

The key to the positive and negative effects of anabolic steroids, including testosterone, is the dose. In biologically normal doses, testosterone increases the libido, improves muscle size and strength, and elevates mood; but in excessive doses, it causes size reduction of the testes, retention of water, and, in women, masculinization. Anabolic steroids in appropriate dosage improves muscle strength and maintenance, but in excessive dosage can cause an unacceptably aggressive personality and physical abnormalities like liver and heart disease.

The usual dose of the most commonly used, long-acting testosterone is 50 to 400 milligrams every two to four weeks. The dose of anabolic steroids for conventional use is variable. For example, the dose of Danozal (Danocrine) is 200 to 800 milligrams daily, taken orally; Stanozol (Winstrol) is 6 milligrams daily taken orally.

In such therapeutic doses, the muscle-building effects of steroids can be achieved without the life-threatening complications, so dosage is a very important determinant in achieving the desired effects without doing harm. Unfortunately, however, many body builders are not satisfied with the slower and less dramatic response of safe doses. They choose the supraphysiological (more than is healthy) doses that create the bulging, ego-stroking muscles. The medical literature is replete with details of overdosing on anabolic steroids. There are descriptions of oral and injected doses of ten to forty times the conventional amounts. The injectable steroids are used in veterinary doses, that is, doses big enough for a horse. Some users dose themselves more than once a day. Others practice "stacking," taking more than one kind of steroid or using increasing doses. A source of problematic steroid use is the many illegal steroids smuggled in from other countries and sold at a great profit. One medical article reports forty-five different varieties on the black market, some of which contain detrimental contaminants. The steroid black market distributes orally administered drugs such as Danozal (Danocrine), Fluoxymesterone (Halotestin), methandrostenolone (Dianabol), oxandrolone

(Anovar), and stanozolol (Winstrol); and injectable drugs like Nandrolone deconoate (Deca-Durobalin) and nandrolone phenpropionate (Durabolin).

By contrast, excessive dosing with testosterone is not a problem because it is provided by prescription only and there are decades of experience behind the dosage selection. Therefore, virtually no black market sale of testosterone exists.

Safe Alternatives to Anabolic Steroids

A person can build strength and endurance in safer ways than using anabolic steroids. Vigorous physical activity is of great benefit. An enormous collection of scientific research clearly demonstrates the value of muscular activity in maintaining healthy bodies and minds.

No one exercise is best for everyone, but the aerobic type is the most valuable. This variety includes walking, jogging, running, bicycling, and swimming. Walking at a fast pace comes the closest to being the perfect exercise for almost everyone, because it is easy, inexpensive, and poses little risk of injury. Probably the best exercise for any individual is simply that which he or she enjoys the most. Weight training also has some value for everyone, even for those in their later years. Some cite the benefits to justify heavy-duty weight lifting, and here is where the trouble starts. It is human nature to believe "if a little is good, a lot is better." When weight lifting is pushed beyond the appropriate levels, muscle, ligament, or tendon injury may occur.

Men who have small muscle mass and are not willing to undergo the rigors of weight training may pursue another physical activity, such as running, to develop strength and endurance. Good endurance is an alternative physical achievement to large muscles.

The body needs protein to sustain and increase muscle mass. Adequate protein intake is also necessary for healthy bones because the matrix containing calcium compounds is composed mostly of protein material.

Proteins are composed of amino acids. Many amino acid preparations are promoted for various purposes, especially to body builders. Although they are a concentrated source, they are not superior to other natural sources found in a daily diet. The same amino acids are found in meat, eggs, milk, legumes, and plant sources (See the Appendix for a further discussion of protein and amino acid supplements.)

CHAPTER TEN

The Feminine Factor

Women and Testosterone

- **Testosterone and Women's Libido**
- **Changes in Libido After Menopause**
- **Testosterone Replacement for Decreased Libido and Menopause**
- **Testosterone Replacement for Other Medical Conditions**
- **Side Effects of Testosterone Treatment**
- **Women Athletes and the Use of Testosterone and Steroids**

Women's bodies produce small amounts of male hormones in their ovaries, adrenals, and other tissues, which in turn are necessary for making the hormones estrone and estradiol. These masculine hormones normally are balanced by a woman's estrogen. Until recently, very little research had been done on the effects of testosterone on women. The most widely known effect is the powerful influence it has on a woman's libido.

Testosterone and Women's Libido

Does testosterone make women feel sexy? Testosterone is indeed a powerful aphrodisiac for women. For many years physicians have prescribed testosterone and other masculinizing hormones to suppress the growth of certain cancers in women. But now women are beginning to use testosterone to enhance their sexuality.

The effects of the male hormones on women are both psychological and physiological. The most noticeable psychological response to more testosterone in the female body is an increased libido, regardless of the woman's libido level before testosterone use. Women's interest in sex is greater. Thoughts of a sexual nature are frequent, intense, and pervasive. Women experience that indescribable feeling of need for sexual gratification, saying that they "want to be loved" or "feel horny." Sex becomes a more important part of their lives and provides more enjoyment, with improved sexual activity, satisfaction, pleasure, and orgasms. Various diseases can impair body functions, including libido, such as diabetes, chronic infections, adrenal or pituitary gland dysfunction, heart disease, and various other disabling conditions. A low libido can be a disrupting force to a relationship, and when significant disparity between a couple's libidos occurs, it can be a source of contention. Usually when this problem exists, a loving, congenial discussion can be an adequate and appropriate means to finding a solution. Both partners must be willing to make concessions and arrive at a mutually acceptable level of sexual activity.

A low libido level may also be the result of a woman who no longer finds her sexual partner attractive or who is involved in a sexually dysfunctional relationship, such as one in which the man may be suppressing a homosexual or asexual preference. In some cases, professional counseling is recommended to resolve these difficulties.

Regardless of age, women's libido increases if testosterone is administered. For some women, increased libido may be a welcome development both to them and their partners. For other women, increased libido can be something of a disaster, as when no sexual partner is available or when the partner has a low libido or is asexual. This circumstance can lead to extramarital sexual activity, or at least a fear of it, by either the woman herself or her spouse. Women who have no access to a sexual partner usually resort to masturbation as a means of relieving sexual cravings. And for women who believe that coitus is sinful, disgraceful, or dirty, a strong urge for sexual activity can be very disturbing.

Changes in Libido after Menopause

After menopause, the adrenals continue to make male hormones, causing a relative increase in testosterone as compared to estrogen. For most women, this hormonal imbalance will lead to some increase in libido around the time of their menopause. Masculinizing effects can also arise when testosterone increases, resulting in symptoms such as increased male pattern hair growth.

Since postmenopausal women continue to secrete small amounts of testosterone from their atrophic ovaries and adrenal glands, their libidos remain at a fairly high level. This can present a problem to a heterosexual couple if the man's libido is diminished due to testosterone deficiency or andropause (see Chapter 7). These couples can often benefit from counseling to understand this disparity in their libidos and learn how to make adjustments about the frequency of sexual activity. Treatment may include testosterone replacement therapy for the man if appropriate.

Testosterone Replacement for Decreased Libido and Menopause

Occasionally testosterone is prescribed in combination with estrogen. The combination may be useful to retard osteoporosis for women at high risk for this condition or women needing a boost in their libido, much as testosterone replacement therapy does for men. For some women sensing a temporarily low libido, a testosterone injection on an as-needed basis might be helpful.

Some physical abnormalities are also associated with lower levels of sexuality. Hypothyroidism (low output of thyroid hormone) has a slowing effect on every organ and cell in the body, so sexuality may be decreased. Depression in both men and women often manifests as a decreased libido as one of the more general symptoms of declining enthusiasm for previously enjoyed activities.

When a physician is unable to detect any other explanation for a low libido, a psychological explanation other than depression may be considered. Testosterone may be part of reasonable and ethical treatment in this situation. Physicians use the terms *therapeutic* or *diagnostic trial* to refer to prescribing a medication for a suspected abnormality and following the patient's response. If, on follow-up visits, the patient reports improvement, the therapeutic trial is deemed successful. A favorable response helps confirm the suspected diagnosis.

It is also suggested that testosterone increases the beneficial effects of estrogen on menopausal symptoms: controlling hot flashes, slowing the atrophy of the vagina, lowering cholesterol and triglyceride levels, slowing of bone demineralization, and reducing sexual dysfunction. Because estrogen is so effective, has other side benefits, and is a natural way to treat women, physicians have had no incentive to replace it altogether with testosterone.

In her popular book, *The Hormone of Desire*, Susan Rako, M.D., promotes the use of estrogen and testosterone combinations. She lists these symptoms as indicating a need for testosterone combinations: low libido, reduced energy and feeling of well-being, lowered sensitivity of the clitoris and nipples, and decreased arousability and capacity for orgasm.

The most commonly prescribed combinations of estrogen and testosterone are Premarin 0.625 (with five milligrams of Methyltestosterone) and Premarin 1.25 (with ten milligrams of Methyltestosterone). Both contain relatively small doses of testosterone. Premarin with testosterone has varying popularity among prescribing physicians. The dose must be kept low because in higher oral doses, testosterone occasionally causes liver disease.

Testosterone Replacement
for Other Medical Conditions

Relatively little research has been conducted regarding testosterone's effects on women. A search of the medical literature reveals only a few studies, including some reporting a positive male hormonal effect in slowing the development of osteoporosis. Adding testosterone to estrogen is more effective than estrogen alone in the control of mineral loss from bones. It could be expected that testosterone alone would also slow osteoporosis in women, but it is not currently being used for that purpose.

A combination of testosterone and estrogen has also been used to effectively treat panhypopituitarism (a congenital female condition in which pubic hair does not develop in pubescent girls) without side effects.

Most of the available and reliable information about the response of women to testosterone is from observing how women's bodies respond to hormone-secreting tumors. Rarely occurring tumors of the ovaries produce large amounts of male hormones and secrete them into the bloodstream. The entire body as well as the psyche respond to the rising hormone blood levels.

Healthy ovaries have special cells that manufacture two male sex hormones. Normally, other cells convert the hormones to estrogen, but some ovarian tumors produce a large excess of these male hormones, which has a masculinizing effect on the female body. The most common of these tumors is the arrhenoblastoma, which is usually a benign tumor. The first sign of the tumor is the stopping of menses, followed by excessive hair growth on the face, acne, shrinking of the breasts, an enlarged clitoris, balding, and a deepening of the voice. In this condition, the woman's blood concentration of testosterone reaches up into the range of a healthy adult male. The body changes cannot be reversed by administering estrogen. When the tumor is surgically removed, menses returns and the abnormal hair growth subsides.

Occasionally, testosterone-related chemicals are given to women for the management of breast cancer. This counteracts the effects of estrogen. Testosterone has never been used as a primary treatment of breast cancer, but rather to slow the metastasis (spread) as well as the growth of the tumor in the breast itself. It has been effective in controlling breast malignancy in two settings. One is when the cancer has advanced beyond the point where treatment is curative, for example, when metastases occur. The other is when traditional treatments such as surgery or radiation are not practical for a patient who has other life-limiting conditions such as advanced heart disease, disabling strokes, or kidney disease.

In the past, testosterone itself was administered to breast cancer patients. Now drugs are available that are modifications of testosterone, with a greater suppressant effect on the tumor and fewer undesirable effects. These are testosterone analogs.

When physicians prescribe a masculinizing hormone for the treatment of a malignancy, they must frankly discuss the side effects with the patient as well as her partner so that they will both be more prepared to cope with the sudden increase in her libido. If increased libido is acceptable to the patient and her mate, no change in medication is needed. If the increase in libido is a problem, her physician can adjust the dose or change to some other form of cancer therapy.

Side Effects of Testosterone Treatment

If it is apparent that testosterone is the appropriate treatment for a woman, it must be given judiciously under a limited dosage schedule to avoid undesired side effects. Dosages in the range near those produced by the adrenals and ovaries skirt this problem. Accordingly, the woman's general health and specifically possible masculinization must be monitored. The masculinizing effects on women are essentially the same as those seen in boys when they enter manhood. New hair growth appears on the face, chest, back, lower abdomen, and inner thighs. The fine soft hair, called vellus hairs, becomes coarse and pigmented. A related change is increased activity of the sebaceous (oil) glands that can cause acne. Hair loss of a male balding pattern and voice deepening may also occur.

When women receive excessively large testosterone doses, there is a detrimental effect on their lipid profile that entails higher levels of triglycerides and LDL ("bad" cholesterol) and lower levels of HDL ("good" cholesterol). Testosterone in very large doses can also block the pituitary hormone's effects on the ovaries so they stop making estrogen. Just as heavy use of testosterone shrinks the testes, it will shrink and inactivate the ovaries and disrupt the menstrual cycle, which can lead to female menopause and/or infertility.

Testosterone administration also causes enlargement of the clitoris in inconsistent degrees from one woman to the next. This increased size is rarely a problem. If the patient is advised of the probable change before beginning therapy with testosterone, it should not be a source of distress. The size of a clitoris is not related to the degree of sensitivity. The enlargement occurs because the clitoris is the female's analogous organ to the penis.

Women Athletes
and the Use of Testosterone and Steroids

It is widely known that estrogen levels can decrease when women become more physically active (weight training, endurance running), resulting in reduced ovarian function. When women use anabolic steroids, their ovaries become inactive. Anabolic steroids have a positive effect on the body's nitrogen balance and so are considered muscle builders. These medications were originally introduced to the medical profession for use on chronically ill patients with wasting diseases like cancer and some chronic infections. This use corresponds to men taking testosterone to retard the aging effect on muscle weakening and shrinkage.

Female body builders use testosterone and, more often, anabolic steroids to strengthen and enlarge their muscles. These substances are effective for this purpose but have some side effects, just as they do for men who use them in large doses (see Chapter 3). Some charlatans are administering or prescribing testosterone for women with a promise of miraculous results. Naturally, this is to be discouraged.

CHAPTER ELEVEN

Looking Ahead

The Future of
Testosterone Research

- The Role of Testosterone in Cognition
- Testosterone Replacement and Osteoporosis
- Tesosterone Replacement for Other Medical Disorders
- New Forms of Testosterone Administration
- New Medications for Impotence
- Chemical Creams for Sexual Difficulties
- Medical Ethics and Testosterone Use
- Conclusion

We have reason to expect an acceleration in testosterone research and an expansion in the application of new knowledge for the management of testosterone deficiency. Diagnostic techniques and skills will undoubtedly improve, understanding will grow about the significance of test results, and physicians will develop a better grasp of what levels of testosterone constitute an abnormality and when treatment is indicated. Medical research will help further define the exact doses needed and result in a more thorough understanding of the side effects of testosterone replacement.

The current medical and pharmaceutical research on testosterone and related testosterone deficiency symptoms in men shows great promise. There is an enormous need for research that can tell physicians when testosterone is useful and advisable for men who would benefit from replacement therapy even when their blood testosterone levels are within normal range (for the use of the hormone in other than those who have a frank deficiency). It would be helpful to have indicators in addition to the blood tests that would delineate when testosterone might enhance the quality of life for men regardless of age. Just as physicians use a woman's expression of low energy, lessened libido, depressed mood, anxiety, and irritability to determine that estrogen replacement might be in order, similar symptomatic indicators should be used to suggest the need for testosterone replacement in men. Until such indicators are recognized in the medical literature, most physicians will be reluctant to prescribe testosterone except when blood test results show an unequivocally low level of the hormone.

The Role of Testosterone in Cognition

No hard evidence is available regarding the effect of testosterone on cognition, but the information we do have is encouraging, though anecdotal. Most people are aware of improved mental acuity when they're happy. On days when everything goes well, their minds are clearer and their memories are intact. It is possible that testosterone will be shown to have a direct effect on some parts of the brain that lead to an improved overall sense of well-being. One study suggests the hippocampus in the brain has receptors for estrogen, so possibly evidence of testosterone receptors will also be found.

It has never been clear whether the differences in male and female cognition are due to the organizing effects of sex hormones at the fetal stage or the activation of the sex hormones in adults. One study found that administering androgens to adult women clearly increased their spatial ability performance while decreasing their verbal fluency. The changes were long lasting. In general, men are able to perform spatial tasks better than women, and women are more verbally skilled than men. There appears to be little question that this difference emerges from the chemical action of the sex hormones on the brain.

Other studies on women's brains demonstrate that estrogen, which is chemically very similar to testosterone, may lessen the damage of strokes, enhance motor function, increase attention, reduce forgetfulness, and promote connections between brain cells in postmenopausal women. One dramatic discovery is that estrogen improves memory and attention in older women with Alzheimer's disease.

Some research has been conducted and reported in the medical literature and at medical meetings on how estrogen affects a woman's mind and intellect. The results are encouraging. It appears that women have greater thinking capacity and memory when taking supplemental estrogen. A recent study reported that the onset of Alzheimer's disease is delayed in women taking estrogen, however, the design of the research has been criticized. The findings may not hold up to close scientific scrutiny.

Because of similar chemical structure and pharmacological effects, it is reasonable to suggest that testosterone might have parallel effects on a man's cognition and memory. Dr. John E. Morley, professor of gerontology at the St. Louis School of Medicine, reported at the Endocrine Society that evidence suggests that testosterone loss may play a role in some form(s) of age-related memory dysfunction and that testosterone supplementation could prove useful for improving men's memory. An expansion of the knowledge base concerning the effects of testosterone on the mind would be very useful to practicing clinicians.

Testosterone Replacement and Osteoporosis

In women we know the first five or ten years of estrogen deficiency is when most of the bone loss occurs. Although estrogen is used to retard osteoporosis, no hard research shows that it actually reverses bone loss related to menopause. Two new products, a nasal spray and a tablet, cause bone replacement in osteoporotic women by slowing normal resorption activity that goes on as bone is in a constant state of breakdown (resorption) and replacement. Research is continuing to determine the use of estrogen with one of these medications.

No current investigation is being made into the use of these products with testosterone for osteoporotic men, but testosterone has also been shown to have a beneficial effect on women's bones. The amount of collagen, a protein that is the main constituent of connective tissue in bones, increased significantly in postmenopausal women treated with a combination of testosterone and estradiol.

Testosterone Replacement for Other Medical Disorders

In men, testosterone testing has yielded positive results for treating prepubescent boys afflicted with constitutionally delayed puberty. All boys treated with intramuscular injections of testosterone entered normal puberty after the treatments.

HIV-positive men also benefit from testosterone replacement therapy. Testosterone administration improves their mood, energy, appetite, and sexual interest and function within eight weeks of starting the therapy.

New Forms of Testosterone Administration

In addition to the skin patches, another new route of administrating testosterone is being studied—long-acting, slow-release microcapsules. In men with low testosterone levels, the microcapsules raised their testosterone levels quickly and maintained it consistently in the mid-normal range for an average of ten weeks. Inserted under the skin by a physician, the microcapsules are easier to use than patches (which have to be applied daily) and are an improvement over even the long-term testosterone injections (which last a few weeks with a fluctuating level of testosterone). However, the Food and Drug Administration (FDA) has yet to approve the microcapsules.

New Medications for Impotence

In 1996, the medical literature reported a new pill for treating male impotence, sildenafil (Pfizer, the manufacturer of the drug, has named it Viagro). The medication is taken orally and reaches maximum blood level within one hour. The onset of effects is also within one hour, but some men have reported responding in as little as fifteen minutes.

The trials of sildenafil have been conducted on men who have psychologically caused impotence. However, some unpublished reports suggest there may be beneficial effects for some men with organic (physical) abnormalities as well. Success rates run as high as 97 percent for psychogenic cases and 80 percent for all cases. In clinical trials there was no change in blood pressure, pulse, or the tested blood chemicals, and the side effects reported were transient: headaches, skin flushing, dyspepsia, and muscle aches.

If and when sildenafil becomes available for general use depends on the results of further research and FDA approval. The present plan is to file for approval by the FDA.

Another naturally produced chemical, the vasorestrictive agent endothelin, is responsible for keeping the penis rigid. It may be possible in the future to inject endothelin directly to maintain erections or to administer a substance that will regulate its release in the body.

Chemical Creams for Sexual Difficulties

Creams are pharmaceutical preparations that are a semisolid emulsion of oil and water. By themselves, they are usually inert but can be used as a vehicle to bring active ingredients (medications) to the skin surface where the medication is absorbed into or through the skin. Some drugs are absorbed better than others. Among those that penetrate the skin and are well absorbed into the bloodstream are the sex hormones, estrogen and testosterone.

One of the problems facing developers of local application preparations containing active ingredients, including testosterone, is how to control the dosage. What one man may consider a small dose, another may consider a large dose. It's human nature to think that if a little is good, a lot is better. One way suggested to regulate dosage is to dispense the cream or lotion in a container that releases a measured dose with each activation, much like bronchodilator canisters do for the control of asthma; with each activation, a certain number of milligrams are delivered. With the growing interest and enthusiasm by patients and practitioners for using testosterone, it would not be surprising if enterprising manufacturers create such a product in the near future.

Testosterone Creams

At the time of this writing, no approved pharmaceutical cream products containing the sex hormones are available. A market exists, however, for creams containing testosterone. It is one of the many drugs that people have access to even though the drug does not have FDA approval. Inasmuch as these creams are "black market" products and do not have FDA recognition, there is no published data or research reports on their use. The people who use these preparations give anecdotally glowing reports of their effectiveness, especially with scrotal applications. As might be expected, their testimonials list the same benefits that are reported for the use of ethically distributed testosterone injections and patches.

The use of testosterone cream on human skin is not entirely without precedence. For many years clinicians have been prescribing testosterone in a cream vehicle for *Lichen sclerosis et atrophicus,* an annoying, chronic skin condition. It is most commonly located on the vulva of women and is a cause of dyspareunia (painful intercourse). Because of its effectiveness in controlling this very troublesome condition, testosterone cream is prescribed by clinicians who treat gynecological conditions even though it has not been approved for this abnormality by the FDA. Pharmacists prepare the cream as directed by the physician on a prescription.

Creams for Erection Difficulties

The *British Medical Journal,* in June 1996, reported research on a skin cream that stimulates penile erections. It was tested on men experiencing impotence due to psychogenic causes, neurological causes, or artery insufficiency. Some men had more than one cause. It was a double-blind cross-over study so that neither the patient nor the doctor knew whether each man was receiving the cream containing the active or inactive ingredient. This eliminated the placebo effect that could invalidate the findings. Fifty-eight percent had satisfactory erections using the cream as compared with 8 percent using the placebo. Even more impressive was the 82 percent rate for those having psychogenic impotence.

The active ingredients are three chemicals known to penetrate the skin and affect artery activity: aminophylline, isosorbide, and a mixture of ergot substances (alkaloids that stimulate the contraction of smooth muscles). Isosorbide is well known to many cardiac patients who take it orally or through skin patches to improve heart function. Ergot products have been used for decades to control vascular headaches such as migraines.

In the tests, neither the patients nor their partners had any side effects, but its use presents some problems; the dosage is difficult to control, for example. With additional research and FDA approval, this product may become available in the United States. Black market creams have already been reported in some locations.

Medical Ethics and Testosterone Use

Testosterone replacement therapy can significantly improve the quality of men's lives. Although most of this book addresses the use of testosterone therapy for men who clearly have a deficiency of the hormone, a big question remains: does testosterone benefit men whose blood tests do not indicate a deficiency but have one or more of the symptoms of testosterone deficiency (men who develop progressive muscle weakness or a low libido or who have lost their feeling of well-being)? Researchers have not yet adequately explored or answered this question.

The medical literature discourages inappropriate use of testosterone therapy but is not clear on what constitutes appropriate or inappropriate use. Practicing clinicians are left to make the decision individually about who should or should not receive the hormone.

Many men hear or read of the wonderful—indeed, miraculous—effects of testosterone on those who have the hormone deficiency. They also hear from men who are not deficient but who, because of the placebo effect, had a perceived revitalization. After hearing these reports and not knowing whether they are deficient, they seek therapy hoping for the same results.

There are two extreme schools of thought on the use of testosterone for aging men. Dr. Eric Orwell, an endocrinologist, represents one side of the issue: "At present, and until more is known concerning the risks and benefits, the routine use of androgen supplements in normal, aging men is probably inappropriate."

On the other extreme are the many reports in the media describing the impressive improvements in the lives of older men using testosterone. This position is predominantly supported by the physicians who prescribe testosterone for their patients but who have not published reports supporting the claims for the arbitrary use of the hormone.

The answer as to who should have testosterone therapy lies somewhere between these two extremes and will be supported in the medical literature in the future. The empirical use of testosterone is ethical and can be justified providing certain criteria are met:

1. The patient must clearly understand that this is a therapeutic trial.

2. Both the patient and the physician must have a realistic concept of what the benefits might be.

3. Both the patient and physician must have a realistic concept of what undesirable side effects might occur.

4. A complete medical evaluation must precede the start of therapy.

5. The patient must indicate a willingness to undergo regular monitoring.

6. The patient must understand the therapy will be discontinued at the physician's discretion based on the development of undesired side effects or failure of the therapeutic trial.

7. The provider must not use unethical advertising promoting the therapy.

8. The provider must not derive financial compensation beyond reasonable and customary fees.

9. The provider must not seek notoriety.

10. The patient must agree to a change in the therapy, including discontinuance, if new scientific information warrants the change.

Conclusion

As physicians and their patients become more aware of testosterone deficiency and the benefits of replacement therapy, the demand will grow for improved methods of introducing the hormone into the body. Estrogen patches for women have proved an efficient means of administering hormones and have received general acceptance by women and their physicians. There is reason to believe testosterone patches will receive similar acceptance. There is also need for a chemical that will provide all of the benefits of testosterone, and at the same time, be effective and safe for swallowing. Such developments will mean that some day testosterone usage will be as common as that of estrogen replacement and will provide similar benefits in the quality of life for men.

CHAPTER TWELVE

Answers to Frequently Asked Questions

What is testosterone?

Testosterone is the principal male sex hormone, made by the testes and responsible for inducing and maintaining primary and secondary male sexual characteristics.

What is a hormone?

It's a chemical produced by certain organs and glands that circulates in body fluids, stimulates cellular activity, and has regulatory effects on other organs.

What are male sex hormones?

They are hormones that have a masculinizing effect all through life, beginning in the embryo. From puberty onward, the sex hormones influence male sexual behavior.

What are the male primary sexual characteristics?

They are formation and enlargement of the external genital structures (the penis and scrotum), and the internal male organs (the prostate and seminal vesicles).

What are some of the male secondary sex characteristics?

They include voice change, growth of body and facial hair, muscle enlargement, and male sexual behavior.

Where in the male body is testosterone produced?

Ninety-five percent of all testosterone is produced by the testes, but a small amount is also made by the adrenal glands.

What other sex hormones do the testes produce?

They produce dihydrotestosterone (a potent, active form of testosterone) and DHEA (a weaker masculinizing hormone). The testes also secrete small amounts of the female hormones, estrogen and progesterone.

How are anabolic steroids related to male sex hormones?

Testosterone is one of the anabolic steroids. Many other anabolic steroids that are chemically similar to testosterone are synthetically produced and used to strengthen muscles, mostly in body builders and athletes.

Is testosterone ever prescribed for its anabolic effect?

Usually not, because it is a relatively weak anabolic steroid and much stronger synthetic anabolic steroids are available for muscle building that don't have the masculinizing side effects of testosterone. The distribution of testosterone is also more rigidly controlled than the synthetic anabolic steroids.

What are the most common side effects of anabolic steroids?

The most pervasive side effects are psychological and include aggressive and sometimes inappropriate behavior. Physical side effects include the shrinkage of the testes and infertility. Anabolic steroid use rarely causes liver disease or heart conditions.

What conditions can cause testosterone deficiency?

It can be caused by some very rare congenital disorders that become apparent in childhood or during puberty, occasionally mumps that involve the gonads, or an extensive injury to both testes.

What are the common causes of testosterone deficiency?

By far the most common reason for testosterone deficiency is gonad insufficiency due to aging changes that reduce the blood flow through the arteries. When the organs, including the testes, receive less blood, the tissues have less oxygenation and chemicals for their nutrition, so they are less efficient.

Does circulation reduction to the testes occur in all men?

Yes, but the process has its onset earlier in life for some men than others, and the rate of arterial change varies from one man to another.

Why do some peoples' arteries age earlier or later than others?

This happens partly because of hereditary characteristics and partly because of general health factors such as blood lipid abnormalities, thyroid disease, or diabetes.

Do any measures reduce the chance of developing testosterone deficiency?

Yes. Adopt a healthy lifestyle early in life and stay with it. Preventative measures include eating a balanced diet, staying active, and avoiding the use of tobacco. It also helps to have regular health assessments to detect artery damaging conditions early so that appropriate corrective measures can be taken.

Is male menopause, or andropause, the same as testosterone deficiency?

No. Although the two conditions share some similar symptoms, andropause is a psychological condition, whereas testosterone is a physical condition. The treatments for the two disorders are entirely different.

Is testosterone deficiency in men parallel to estrogen deficiency, or menopause, in women?

They are similar in that they both are caused by the gonads producing less hormone, but estrogen deficiency happens abruptly, occurs in all women in midlife, and results in sterility, while testosterone deficiency happens very gradually, over decades, is not universal in all men, and rarely results in sterility.

Why is testosterone prescribed for women?

It is occasionally prescribed, in much smaller doses than men take, to increase libido.

What side effects do women have when using male hormones?

Facial and body hair grow, the clitoris enlarges, and some women develop more masculine body contours, including shrinking breasts. Occasionally the voice deepens, menses may stop, and the woman may become sterile.

What are the physical symptoms of testosterone deficiency?

Any time after puberty, the signs may include a lower libido, impotence, low energy, or a decrease in body and facial hair. In the more severe cases, the muscles decrease in size, resulting in weakness.

What are the psychological symptoms of testosterone deficiency?

Apathy can appear as a manifestation of the reduced energy. This may masquerade as a clinical depression. Sometimes family members notice increased irritability.

What should a man do if he suspects he may be experiencing testosterone deficiency?

He should consult his physician.

How is testosterone deficiency diagnosed?

A doctor takes a medical history, asks health questions, and does a physical examination that includes the external genitalia and the prostate. If there is reason to suspect a testosterone deficiency, the doctor can order blood tests that might include a testosterone level determination and possibly other hormone concentrations in the blood. Tests for evidence of some other condition to explain the symptoms, such as diabetes or thyroid disease, may also be ordered.

What are the treatment options if testosterone deficiency is confirmed?

Generally, gonad insufficiency, the cause of testosterone deficiency, is irreversible, so the treatment is usually testosterone replacement therapy. The treatment options are (1) to treat or not to treat and (2) which testosterone administration method to use—injections, skin patches, or some other delivery route.

What does testosterone therapy cost?

Prices vary depending on the method of testosterone administration. At this time, the long-lasting injections cost about $8 a month, the shorter-duration injections are about $50 a month, and testosterone patches from the pharmacy run about $80 to $100 a month.

Are there any side effects from testosterone replacement therapy?

Significant side effects are minimal. Less that 5 percent of patients experience mild headaches, indigestion, or allergic reactions. A few patients develop a rash or itching at either the scrotal or nonscrotal skin sites where the patches are applied.

What is the first noticeable benefit from replacement therapy?

Men notice a feeling of increased well-being generally sense after a few days of testosterone therapy.

How soon will sexual function improve after starting treatment?

Because the sense of well-being improves, and sometimes due to the placebo effect, sexual function can start improving in two to three days. For the actual physiological and pharmacological improvements to take effect, a longer period of time is needed. The average time for an improvement in libido is three to six months. Resolution of an impotence problem may take longer.

What are the long-term physical benefits of replacement therapy?

Testosterone reduces the number of bone fractures in later life. By improving the calcium balance in the boncs, it reduces osteoporosis. It also helps the muscles remain healthier, and there is less loss of muscle size and strength when taking testosterone.

Is there any danger of getting prostate cancer from testosterone replacement therapy?

No scientific evidence indicates that testosterone causes cancer of the prostate, but when prostate cancer is already present, testosterone makes the tumor grow faster and become more difficult to control.

How is a patient protected against the complications of increased prostate cancer growth while using replacement therapy?

Before initiating therapy, the physician checks to determine whether there is any evidence of prostate cancer. Patients on testosterone therapy have their prostates checked regularly by their physician, usually at six-month intervals.

How does the doctor check for prostate cancer?

By examining the prostate with a finger in the rectum, a physician can determine whether there is prostate growth, irregularities, or lumps. In addition, a doctor analyzes a blood test for the prostate-specific antigen (PSA) level in the blood.

Is it true that the PSA is not completely reliable in detecting prostate cancer?

A single blood test for PSA is less reliable than tests for some other cancers, but when PSA is tested regularly, a rising level over a number of tests can indicate the possibility of cancer.

What happens if the PSA goes up during testosterone therapy?

The testosterone treatment is immediately discontinued. Additional testing by biopsy or imaging studies may be scheduled. Prostate cancer diagnosis and management are essentially the same for men who have been using testosterone replacement as for those who have not.

What future benefits can be expected from research into the medical use of testosterone?

Studies are being directed at finding better sources of testosterone and better delivery systems—related chemicals that have the same benefits with fewer side effects and improved methods of administration. Some clinicians believe testosterone replacement will become much more widely used, approaching the use of estrogen for menopause.

CHAPTER THIRTEEN

Doc Talk

Information for Physicians

- **Assessing Low Libido and Impotence**
- **Diagnosing Testosterone Deficiency**
- **Assessment of Testosterone Deficiency**

- **Laboratory Testing**
- **Monitoring and Evaluating Testosterone Replacement Therapy**
- **Drugs and Sexual Dysfunction**

Few men suffering with sexual problems will seek help from their doctors or volunteer this information unless asked directly about it. Unfortunately, most physicians don't ask, although more medical schools are now teaching courses on sexuality. The number of articles in medical journals about the importance of male sexual health has increased significantly in the past ten years, which has helped men become slightly less reluctant to discuss their sexual shortcomings and concerns.

If both the partners are under the care of the same physician, then that physician is in a good position to assist them in improving their sexual relationship and sometimes their emotional relationship as well. The physician must use extreme tact and be verbally nimble in handling the problem. Management of the physical condition is fairly easy and straightforward, but management of the psychological aspects are more challenging. It can be difficult, but the reward of knowing that a couple has responded positively to treatment makes the effort worthwhile.

Assessing Low Libido and Impotence

When a physician sees a man who is concerned about sexual dysfunction, the first question he or she should very tactfully ask is how the patient feels about his sexual partner. Only occasionally will a man offer unsolicited information about his feelings for his wife or significant other. If artfully done, a starting point some physicians use is to ask, "Do you love your wife?" The answer may be long in coming. The patient may be forced, for the first time in years, to come to grips with how he actually feels. A less threatening question may be, "How do you feel about your wife? Does she turn you on?"

A man's sexual partner is often the first to notice the symptoms of waning libido. Women's sexuality does not significantly decrease during or after menopause. If sexual activity becomes less frequent, she generally becomes aware of her husband's sexual slowdown. Men seldom come to the doctor's office with a chief complaint of lower libido, but given an opening by the physician they willingly discuss it. When asked directly, "How is your sex drive?" men will respond with something like, "I'm slowing down considerably, but I guess that's to be expected at my age. I really don't seem to need sex as much as when I was younger." The caring and skilled physician will probably then ask, "Is this OK with your wife?" The response will then be either, "Yes, it's OK with her; she tells me she is happy without a sex life," or, "We haven't discussed it, but I'm afraid she would like to have sex a little more often." Discussion of the problem proceeds from there, depending on the answer.

Few men make appointments with their doctors because of impotence. Most make an appointment for some minor ailment and then, during the course of their visit, hint that an erection problem is the real reason for the visit. "Say, Doc, while I'm here, is there something that would help my sex life?" Whether it comes in a "Say, Doc" statement or as a response to a question during a general physical examination, men have a sense of gratitude and relief when invited to discuss their sexual problems. When a man has an appointment for a general health assessment, the doctor should inquire about his sexual function by asking about sexual problems, erections, and orgasms. When erectile dysfunction is the complaint, the investigation to determine the cause begins with questions, followed by a physical examination. The history is the most helpful, for example, in discovering how abrupt the onset of impotence was. If the onset was abrupt, the cause is more likely to be of a psychological nature. Physical causes have a gradual onset.

When the problem of impotence develops over a period of a few days or weeks, the diagnosing physician seeks a psychological explanation. Sometimes the man offers an explanation such as, "It started when my promotion didn't come through," or, "When my wife had pelvic surgery," or, "When I had an extramarital affair at the convention I attended in Las Vegas last year," or "When my ankle was in a cast after the skiing accident last winter." If the man fails to offer his own explanation or triggering event, the physician must ask some appropriate questions. If skilled, a physician can focus in on the emotional event that might have resulted in psychogenic impotence. If the clinician also cares for other members of the patient's family, he or she may already know about an emotionally traumatizing event, such as the divorce of one of the children, a financial reverse, or the death of a friend or relative. Commonly the event involves an unresolved marital problem or an injury or illness the man perceives as being related to his sex organs.

Physicians who suspect low libido or impotence should order testosterone blood levels early in the investigation. They know from experience that it's difficult to correct the problem in the presence of a testosterone deficiency regardless of what other reasons there may be for the erectile dysfunction. The test is accurate, widely available, and not expensive, so it's a good starting point. If the lab tests show that the testosterone blood level is low, additional tests are often needed before a treatment can be correctly selected. More sophisticated testing may be needed to distinguish between hormonal and non-hormonal causes.

Diagnosing Testosterone Deficiency

Men whose bodies are deficient in testosterone have both physical and mental abnormalities. Symptoms from the physical disturbance create or add to the mental unrest. Awareness of deteriorating physical health is psychologically distressing. Angst, depression, and low self-esteem are common responses. These feelings are disrupting to personal relationships and may produce psychosocial problems. The physical changes decrease feelings of well-being. Muscle weakness and impaired sexual function decrease a man's pleasure in life and his concept of his masculinity.

A man may arrive at his physician's office with a variety of complaints or symptoms when he is deficient in testosterone. Usually there is more than one symptom, and the symptoms overlap. Men use vague terms to describe their symptoms, and the onset of their symptoms is gradual; a man often has difficulty pinpointing a date at which they started.

Psychological changes are the most common symptoms of testosterone deficiency. A testosterone-deficient man might report impaired memory by saying, "I just can't remember things and names as well as I used to; I guess I'm getting old." Another common psychological symptom is dysphoria. The man usually doesn't directly say he is unhappy but is more likely to say something like, "I'm not enjoying things as much as I used to. I'm not even enjoying golf like I did. I just don't have much enthusiasm for anything anymore." Usually his doctor has to draw him out with specific questions to help determine whether dysphoria is present.

A lower level of energy, usually associated with angst, is often the first symptom the man presents to his physician. This may be accompanied by a sleep disorder. A man who has to push himself to go to work or start tasks is likely to have some feelings of anxiety, which translates into disruption in his personal relationships. The man who is discontented and anxious becomes irritable and less enjoyable to be around. When this occurs, his partner might bring the symptoms to his or his physician's attention.

Some testosterone-deficient men seek help for weakness. By weakness, they may mean fatigue, decreasing endurance, or actual muscle weakness as indicated by failure to reach goals in fitness activity. The physician must ask appropriate questions to determine just what the patient is referring to as weakness. If it is truly muscle weakness, testosterone deficiency could well be the cause. With a combination of these symptoms, the man often has a reduced self-esteem. He won't verbalize this, but his physician will probably detect it.

Assessment of Testosterone Deficiency

The testes have two primary functions: to produce sperm and to produce testosterone. Sperm are made by tissues of the seminiferous tubules in the gonads, and testosterone is produced by the Leydig cells. The seminiferous tubules are more subject to destructive processes than are the Leydig cells. They are also affected more by radiation, chemicals, trauma, cancer chemotherapy, and viral illnesses than are the Leydig cells. Testosterone levels are not usually affected by chemotherapy for cancer, but mumps or gonorrhea orchitis (inflammation of the testes) affects both the seminiferous tubules and the Leydig cells. Microscopic studies of the aging testes often show patchy degeneration of the seminiferous tubules when the Leydig cells still appear normal. This condition implies a man may be sterile, producing no sperm or fewer than normal sperm, and yet still be making testosterone in normal amounts. The disparity between the damage required to reduce seminiferous tubules and the Leydig cell functions also suggests an explanation of why testes of smaller than average size may still be producing significant amounts of testosterone.

When a man describes symptoms that are compatible with testosterone deficiency, the physician must consider several possibilities before establishing a firm diagnosis. For example, the symptoms of testosterone deficiency and depression are very similar, including lethargy, low energy level, lassitude, dysphoria, sleep disorders, loss of self-esteem, anxiety, and diminished libido. The physician must be very careful not to make a diagnosis of inadequate testosterone before being certain the man is not suffering a true clinical depression. Occasionally, the two conditions will coexist, and both require treatment. Good clinical judgment by the physician is essential to a safe and effective outcome.

In addition to depression, testosterone deficiency can mimic other psychiatric conditions such as anxiety and andropause. Administration of testosterone for these other conditions is of no benefit in these cases, so a correct diagnosis of testosterone deficiency is essential to the treatment plan.

Another possibility to rule out is hypothyroidism. The thyroid is a regulatory gland for all other organs and tissues of the body. It sort of balances the acceleration and braking effect of different parts of the body. Inadequate output of the thyroid hormone has a slowing effect on the metabolism of the body's organs and tissues. In past decades, hypothyroidism was always considered as a cause for obesity. Now it is understood that a person in the hypothyroid state may be at their ideal weight or over- or underweight. In advanced stages, severe hypothyroidism causes the accumulation of a special type of fluid containing a saccharide (a carbohydrate, one of which is sugar). This accumulation causes weight gain but is not due to an increase in fat. Older patients are at high risk for hypothyroidism. Some studies reveal an incidence as high as 10 percent in patients over sixty-five. Some of the symptoms thyroid- and testosterone-deficient patients share are weakness, fatigue, lethargy, decreased memory and mental acuity, decreased libido, and other sexual impairments.

Diabetes mellitus is a notorious cause of impotence. Uncontrolled, diabetes mellitus can damage nerves and arteries. Unfortunately, impotence caused by diabetes mellitus is irreversible, so men should be checked for this disease, especially if there is diabetes mellitus in the family. If diabetes mellitus is found early and controlled, destruction of the nerves and arteries can be retarded.

The physical examination is of limited value in diagnosing testosterone deficiency, but a general examination is of definite benefit for finding other abnormalities that mimic the condition. If no other explanation is found, the diagnostic efforts are directed to gonadal function. The size and firmness of the testes may be significant. Small or soft testes may be consistent with a diagnosis of gonadal deficiency, but exceptions are common. On the other hand, the finding of large, firm testes does not rule out testosterone deficiency. This leaves laboratory testing as the only means of accurately diagnosing testosterone deficiency.

Laboratory Testing

Physicians treating sexual dysfunction should order testosterone blood levels early in the investigation. They know from experience that it's difficult to correct the problem in the presence of a testosterone deficiency regardless of what other reasons there may be for the erectile dysfunction. The test is accurate, widely available, and inexpensive, so it's a good start-ing point.

A normal blood level of testosterone is between 300 and 1,100 nanograms per deciliter, but variation in the normal level has, as yet, not been linked to specific age groups other than before and after puberty. These ballpark figures are not very helpful in determining whether any individual man is deficient in testosterone. Much of a man's circulating testos-terone, up to 30 percent, is bound to the protein albumin, the sex hormone-binding globulin (SHBG). SHBG–bound testos-terone is inactive. It is essentially inert and has no androgenic effect. Thus, the total testosterone can be in the normal range, but the free, active form will be low. Other tables sidestep the question by using the term *reference range* instead of *normal range*. Reference range simply reflects the levels healthy, nor-mal men demonstrate in their blood. This is not very helpful in determining an individual's need for testosterone replace-ment therapy.

Since the range is both broad and variable, it becomes difficult to know whether men with low-normal testosterone levels should be treated. Would they be "healthier" if their testosterone were maintained in the upper range? It would be useful, but not practical, to follow an individual's testos-terone levels from year to year. Knowing that an individual's level ranged from 600 to 900 until the age of fifty-five, then started dropping, a clinician would probably be more likely to prescribe TRT when the level reached 400, even though this is in the normal range by standard measurement. On the other hand, if a man in his sixties is experiencing muscle weakness, low libido, and depression, but his testosterone level is 900, his physician would look elsewhere to explain his symptoms.

Determinations of blood levels of follicle-stimulating hormone (FSH) and luteinizing hormone (LH) are useful for distinguishing the primary cause of low testosterone levels. Another pituitary hormone, prolactin, is sometimes checked because excessive amounts of prolactin from the pituitary gland suppresses testosterone output. This usually happens because of a benign tumor of the pituitary, which is treated with either surgical removal or an oral medication, bromocriptin. SHBG levels are also checked, since this protein attaches to testosterone and renders it unavailable for its androgenic effect. SHBG reportedly increases as one ages, which suggests one reason older men experience less effect from their circulating testosterone. Additional tests can be of some use, but for most cases only the total testosterone test and/or the free testosterone test are needed to select appropriate treatment.

In the past, a urine test was used to determine testosterone levels. The test required saving all of the urine collected over twenty-four hours. Now a blood test is used, and it is much more convenient and accurate. Usually a single blood drawing is adequate, but in some cases a second drawing may be ordered after the results of the first test are available. As with all laboratory tests, it is the physician's responsibility to select a facility in which he has confidence as established by prior experience.

The patient need not fast before the blood drawing, but timing is important. Because of the body's circadian rhythm, the highest level of testosterone occurs around 8:00 in the morning. The intraday variation decreases with advancing age. When the effect of testosterone administration is tested, each drawing should be done at the same time of day, but a physician can interpret the results if he or she knows what time of day the blood was drawn in relation to previous tests. For increased accuracy, the testing should be done in the same lab each time. Blood from one drawing can also be used to test cholesterols, anemias, liver and kidney function, thyroid function, diabetes, and HIV. If these additional tests are to be done, however, the patient should be fasting.

Monitoring and Evaluating Testosterone Replacement Therapy

Part of the monitoring regimen for men using TRT is the blood tests for testosterone levels. Physicians don't agree as to how often this should be done. Early in treatment, the tests are performed more often to assist in adjusting the dose. After the adjustment period, the tests are less frequent. The test is done three to four weeks after initiation of testosterone use, then every three months, and eventually at six-month intervals.

When evaluating the therapeutic trial, the physician and patient should take into consideration the placebo effect. It is sometimes difficult to identify the placebo effect, but most skilled physicians become accurate in recognizing it. The placebo effect may last for a lifetime. Patients seem inclined to say, "Whatever works, use it." Some physicians may agree with these patients. However, as in most of medicine, a good physician does not take the "cookbook approach" to selecting therapy for a patient but rather individualizes the therapy to the specific patient.

Drugs and Sexual Dysfunction

Abnormal sexual function occurs as a side effect with a large number of drugs and medications. The abnormalities are caused by drugs working on the nervous system, the vascular system, and hormone production (see Figure 13-1).

Illegal drugs such as cannabis and heroin are known to lower plasma testosterone levels. Various over-the-counter and prescription drugs lower the libido, others block transmission of nerve messages and interfere with erectile function, and others delay or prevent orgasms.

Tagamet (cimetidine) and other related H_2 receptor blocking drugs that are used for ulcers and other upper digestive tract disorders have antiandrogen effects. Approximately half of the patients taking Tagamet have sexual dysfunction. Tagamet has induced impotence and breast changes in patients with gastric hypersecretory states. It is now sold over the counter as well as in larger-strength tablets by prescription.

Flutamide, a 5-alpha-reductase inhibitor, which is prescribed for control of benign prostate hyperplasia, shows some interesting effects. It increases the level of testosterone but is also associated with decreased libido and impotence because it blocks the access of the testosterone to target cells.

A 36 percent incidence of erectile dysfunction is linked to diuretics, which are commonly used to control high blood pressure.

Beta-adrenoceptor blockers, commonly called beta blockers, are commonly used for hypertension and other cardiovascular treatments. Present-day medical research indicates a beta blocker is the best single drug to reduce the chances of a second heart attack. But these substances, some more than others,

Figure 13-1. Drugs that have all been reported as altering sexual function

	L*	ED	O
Antibiotics			
Ketoconazole		†	
Antidepressants–Tricyclic			
Amitriptyline	†	†	
Amoxapine	†	†	
Clomipramine	†	†	†
Desipramine	†	†	
Doxepin	†		
Imipramine	†		
Maprotiline	†	†	
Protriptyline	†	†	
Trimipramine	†	†	
Antidepressants–Serotonin (5-HT) uptake inhibitors			
Fluoxetine	†	†	†
Paroxitine	†	†	†
Sertraline	†	†	†
Venlafoxine	†	†	†
Antidepressants–Other cyclic agents			
Bupropion	†	†	
Nefazodone	†		
Trazadone	†		
Antidepressants–Mono-amine-oxidase inhibitors			
Phenelzine			†
Transcypromine		†	

*NOTE: L = change in libido; ED = erectile dysfunction; 0 = delayed orgasm or anorgasmia.

(continued)

Figure 13-1. Drugs that have all been reported as altering sexual function

	L*	ED	O
Antihypertension drugs–Diuretics			
Bendroflumethiazine		†	
Chlorthalidone		†	
Chlorothiazide		†	
Hydrochlorothiazide		†	
Polythiazide		†	
Antihypertension Drugs–Beta adrenergic blockers			
Acebutolol	†	†	
Atenolol	†	†	
Betaoxolol	†	†	
Labetolol	†	†	
Metroprolol	†	†	
Nadolol	†	†	
Pindolol	†	†	
Propranolol	†	†	
Sotolol	†	†	
Trinolol	†	†	
Antihypertension drugs–Calcium channel blocking			
Amlodipine		†	
Felodipine	†		
Isradipine	†	†	
Nicardipine		†	
Nifedipine		†	
Verapamil		†	
Antihypertension drugs–Other			
Clonidine		†	
Doxazosin		†	

Figure 13-1. Drugs that have all been reported as altering sexual function

	L*	ED	O
Lobetalol	†	†	†
Methyldopa		†	
Prazosin		†	
Reserpine		†	
Terazosin		†	
Hormones			
Estrogen	†	†	
5-alpha-reductase inhibitors	†	†	
Drugs for indigestion			
Anticholinergics		†	
Histamine H$_2$ receptor antagonist		†	
Narcotics			
Cocaine		†	†
Cannabis (marijuana)		†	†
Heroin		†	†
Methadone	†	†	
Morphine		†	
Sedatives			
Alcohol	†	†	†
Barbituates		†	†
Benzodiazepines	†	†	†
Phenothiazines		†	
Stimulants			
Amphetamines			†
Appetite control drugs	†	†	

are known to interfere with libido and erectile function. The incidence of erectile dysfunction is reported to be 13.8 percent greater using a beta blocker than a placebo.

Physicians are often confronted with a dilemma: what to do when a patient is taking a drug of choice for a particular condition but has a sexual dysfunction that is known to be caused by the drug. If a primary physician is treating both a cardiac condition and sexual dysfunction in the same man, for example, he or she may discuss it with the patient, give the patient appropriate information, and let him make the decision. They may agree to try a less effective drug for the heart condition, one that does not interfere with sexual function. The angiotensin-converting enzyme (ACE) inhibitors are among the few medications used for hypertension that have been found to not contribute to erectile dysfunction, which may account for their popularity. The clinician might also refer the patient for second opinions to two specialists, a psychiatrist or urologist and a cardiologist, and let the specialists handle the two problems separately.

Not all cases require a difficult decision. When the sexual dysfunction is the result of excessive alcohol use, it is easy to advise reducing or ending alcohol intake. If a drug used for the treatment of indigestion such as Tagamet is responsible for sexual dysfunction, many alternative drugs and other treatment methods are available for controlling this condition.

APPENDIX

Overview of the Endocrine System

The wonderful and amazing human body is composed of hundreds of intricate systems. Operating within these systems are thousands of functions ranging from the simple to the complex. To put it into perspective, the most sophisticated computer can duplicate only a handful of body functions, and only those functions that are minimal or basic.

The nervous system and the endocrine system are two examples of intricate body systems. These two systems are important for the way the body communicates or sends messages from one site to another. For this and other reasons, both of these systems play important roles in regard to the sex hormones, sexual development, and sexual behavior. Although the functions of the two systems are related, they use different mechanisms to accomplish their tasks. The information communicated by these two systems helps the body adjust to, and meet the demands of, the environment.

The *nervous system* includes the brain, spinal cord, and peripheral (or outlying) nerves. The nervous system communicates by sending electronic impulses along the nerve cell. As these impulses travel, they must cross the spaces between individual nerve cells (called *synapses*). Chemicals called *neurotransmitters* are the mechanism by which the message crosses the synapse. The action of the nervous system can be characterized as relatively fast.

The *endocrine system* is a network of glands and peripheral tissues (outlying tissues, mostly muscles and fat) that produce chemicals called *hormones*. The endocrine system communicates by secreting hormones into the bloodstream to be carried to another site in the body. There are cells (called *receptor cells*) at the distant site that are capable of reading these hormone "messages." These cells will then carry out some action depending on the presence and concentration of the hormones. In contrast to the workings of the nervous system, the action of hormones on cells is slow, but the effects are long-lasting.

Communication within the endocrine system and the nervous system can sometimes overlap. Some anatomists consider two glands of the endocrine system, the posterior pituitary and the adrenal medulla, to be part of the nervous system. In these glands, nerve impulses can trigger hormone release and vice versa. For example, some chemicals (such as dopamine) can serve as both hormones and neurotransmitters.

The Endocrine System and the Sex Hormones

The endocrine system includes the hypothalamus (a brain structure), the pituitary gland (located in the brain), the adrenal glands (located above the kidneys), the thymus, the pancreas, the thyroid and parathyroid glands, and the reproductive glands (known as *gonads*). The male gonads are the testes; the female gonads are the ovaries.

Controlled by the hypothalamus and pituitary gland, the male gonads (testes) produce a number of male sex hormones (called *androgens*) in addition to making sperm. *Androgen* is a generic term meaning any substance that has a masculinizing effect. Testosterone and its related male sex hormones are considered androgens. The most important androgens are testosterone, dihydrotestosterone (DHT), and estradiol. The other naturally occurring androgens are dehydroepiandrosterone (DHEA), dehydroepiandrosterone sulfate (DHEA[S]), and androstenedione.

The two most important female sex hormones are estrogen and progesterone. *Estrogen* is a generic term that refers to a group of female sex hormones that include estradiol, estrone, and estriol. Estradiol is the most potent; estriol, the least potent. All of these hormones have a feminizing effect. Most estrogens are produced by the ovaries during the first days of the menstrual cycle, but a few are produced by the adrenal glands.

Although progesterone is usually thought of as a female sex hormone, it plays an important role in the hormonal balance of men. The testes produce small amounts of the estrogens as well as progesterone. Progesterone is somewhat more masculine in its effects than estrogen.

The adrenal glands can produce excessive quantities of hormones. Excessive production of sex hormones can cause premature signs of sexual development in very young children or masculine characteristics in women.

The Production of Testosterone

The nervous system actually controls the production of testosterone. Only in recent decades have scientists and physicians appreciated this fact. The hypothalamus (a brain structure) causes the nearby pituitary gland (located in the brain) to make leuteinizing hormone (LH) and follicle-stimulating hormone (FSH). The LH stimulates the testes to produce testosterone, and the FSH stimulates the testes to make sperm. One method of detecting testosterone deficiency is to measure the amount of LH in the blood.

Two other parts of the brain, the cortex and the limbic system, affect the hypothalamus with another hormone called LH-releasing hormone, which is produced by certain brain cells. LH-releasing hormone stimulates the pituitary to release more LH, causing the testes to produce more testosterone.

Ninety-five percent of a man's testosterone is produced in the testes. The remaining 5 percent is made by the adrenal glands. The testes also produce a small amount of the "weak" androgen called dehydroepiandrosterone, popularly referred to as DHEA.

Testosterone is made by the body from cholesterol, in five steps (see Figure A-1): cholesterol > pregnenolone > 17 alpha-hydroxypregnenolone > and dehydroepiandrosterone (DHEA) > androstenediol > testosterone. (The body manufactures its own cholesterol in needed amounts, regardless of the cholesterol ingested. A man cannot affect his testosterone production by dietary manipulation.) Testosterone, like all the other male and female sex hormones, contains carbon, hydrogen, and oxygen atoms. It is the number of these atoms and their arrangement within the molecules that determines their action on the body. In the case of testosterone and estrogen, only slight variations in their chemical structure cause one to be a male sex hormone and the other to be a female sex hormone. This small variation creates a profound difference: one hormone increases facial hair growth, and the other enlarges the breasts.

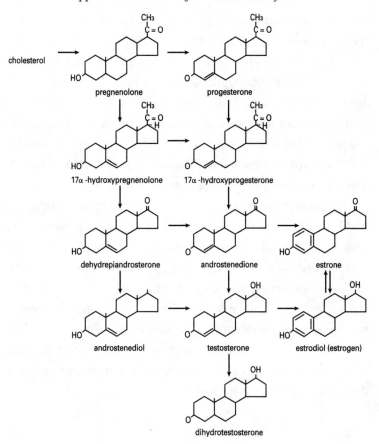

Figure A-1. Chemical synthesis of the androgens and estrogens in men

The Life Cycle of Testosterone

Men produce 2.5 to 10 milligrams of testosterone per day. Approximately 98 percent of the testosterone is bound (or fastened) to protein in the bloodstream. The remaining testosterone is unbound (or free) in the bloodstream. Only the free testosterone is biologically active.

The normal blood plasma concentration of testosterone is 250 to 1,000 nanograms per deciliter. One deciliter is approximately one-fifth of a pint, a nanogram is one-billionth of a gram, and a gram is about one-thirtieth of an ounce. So the amount of circulating testosterone in the blood is minute. It is truly amazing that a man's sexuality can be altered by such a small amount of circulating testosterone.

Testosterone is rapidly broken down by the body. The half-life of testosterone in the body is only ten to twenty minutes, which means that one-half of the body's total testosterone is destroyed by the liver every ten to twenty minutes. Testosterone is converted to other chemicals in the liver (androsterone and etiochololanlone), which are just steps leading to the eventual excretion of testosterone in the urine.

When testosterone is introduced into the body by patch or injection, it acts exactly the same as the testosterone that is naturally produced in the testes.

The Influence of Testosterone on Growth and Development

The male sex hormones are responsible for initiating reproductive functions and developing secondary sex characteristics (such as body hair). They also influence overall growth, body development, and gender-oriented behavior. The male sex hormones regulate both sex drive and potency in men, but they do not determine whether a man is heterosexual or homosexual.

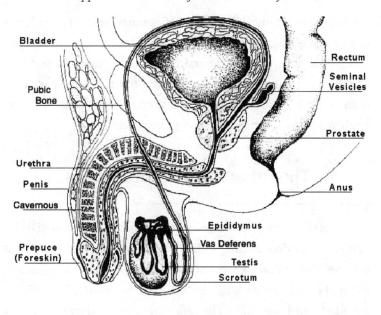

Figure A-2. The adult male genitourinary system

Testosterone levels are relatively high during three periods of the male life cycle. The first is during fetal development, particularly a critical time between the eighth and fourteenth week of gestation when sexual differentiation occurs. Sexual differentiation refers to whether the fetus will develop into a biological male or female. If a sufficient amount of testosterone is present during this time, the growth of internal male genital system structures (the vas deferens, epididymis, and seminal vesicles) will occur (see Figure A-2.) If there is insufficient testosterone, the fetus will continue uninterrupted in its development as a biological female.

The first few months after birth is the second time that a male's testosterone levels are relatively high. Scientists do not yet fully understand the purpose of elevated testosterone levels at this stage of growth. The third time testosterone levels are elevated is during adult sexual life, which begins at puberty. The testosterone levels are low in the prepubescent years (less than 20 nanograms/deciliter) and then increase sharply in the adult years (to 300 to 1,000 nanograms/deciliter).

The Other Male Sex Hormones

The testes secrete testosterone, dihydrotestosterone (DHT), dehydroepiandrosterone sulfate (DHEA[S]), estradiol, and estrone. Peripheral tissues (outlying tissue, mostly muscles and fat) make and secrete testosterone, dihydrotestosterone (DHT), estradiol, and estrone. The adrenal glands secrete the sex hormones dihydrotestosterone (DHT), DHEA, DHEA(S), and androstenedione.

The organs in the body that will be affected by the testosterone circulating in the bloodstream are called *target organs.* As the testosterone leaves the bloodstream, it rapidly crosses the cell membranes of the target organs and enters the plasma inside the cells. Testosterone itself is relatively inactive within the cells of the target organ. Most of the action on the body's cells is due to DHT, so it is considered the most biologically active form of the male sex hormones (the androgens). Nearly all the DHT in the body is produced when testosterone enters the cells of target organs and is changed into DHT by an enzyme. About 20 percent of the body's DHT is made by the adrenal glands.

Once inside the cells, both testosterone and DHT can bind to receptor proteins. The hormones then move from the plasma into the nucleus of the cell. Testosterone and DHT provide androgen action on the cells of target organs by stimulating the synthesis of new protein.

DHT is responsible for the development of the internal and external male genital system (penis and scrotal structures) and the prostate during fetal life. This hormone also controls the growth of the scrotum, epididymis, vas deferens, prostate, and penis during puberty (see Figure A-2). The secondary male sex characteristics, such as muscle growth and the enlargement of the larynx (voice deepening), are also controlled by DHT. This hormone has many of the same effects as testosterone, including the masculinizing effects.

DHT is also of special interest because of its role in prostate enlargement. Benign prostatic hyperplasia (known as BPH) is a common condition that causes urinary bladder symptoms in older men.

The male hormone DHEA functions as a precursor to testosterone production in men. (A *precursor* is a substance from which another substance is synthesized.) Another related hormone, DHEA(S), is also a precursor to the production of testosterone. Both of these hormones occur during the synthesis of testosterone from cholesterol (see Figure A-1). The body actually produces much more DHEA(S) than testosterone. Because DHEA(S) is a "weaker" androgen, using it to increase the overall testosterone level in the body is not the most efficient method. The addition of sulfate to DHEA to create DHEA(S) results in a substance that is more stable in the body and has a longer half-life. (DHEA and DHEA[S] can be used interchangeably in practical discussions, but they are distinguished when needed for scientific purposes.) The chief producers of these hormones are the adrenal glands. Small amounts are also produced by the testes in men and by the ovaries in women. In men, less than 10 percent of DHEA(S) is made by the testes.

By themselves, DHEA and DHEA(S) have "weak" masculinizing effects. If the adrenal glands malfunction, however, these two hormones can produce androgenic effects such as excessive hair growth or the masculinization of a woman's body, though with much less effect than testosterone. Plasma concentrations of DHEA and DHEA(S) peak at about twenty years of age and then decrease progressively with age.

Estrone and estradiol are usually considered female hormones, but they are also part of the chemical synthesis of testosterone (see Figure A-1). They are both made by the testes and the peripheral tissues (outlying tissues, mostly muscle and fat).

Progesterone is usually considered a female hormone that is also produced by males. It affects other organs and tissues by producing changes in carbohydrate, protein, and lipid (fat) metabolism. Because it is less feminizing in its effects than estrogen, some consider it a "weak" androgen.

Scientific Findings on the Use of DHEA and DHEA(S)

(Note: For this practical discussion, DHEA and DHEA[S] can be considered as interchangeable, although they are considered different when viewed from a strictly scientific standpoint.)

Two of the other male sex hormones, dehydroepiandrosterone (DHEA) and dehydroepiandrosterone sulfate (DHEA[S]), have generated some interest among researchers. The scientific research to date on DHEA(S) is scanty, so its use cannot be ethically recommended by practicing physicians at the present time. There is a need for reproducible double-blind studies to either confirm or deny the potential effects of the hormone.

Despite the lack of conclusive scientific evidence, claims are being made in the media and advertising for the benefits of using the other male sex hormones. Some of these as yet unfounded claims for DHEA(S) are that it increases or preserves muscle size, decreases fat, and reduces obesity. There are also unproven statements that it relieves insomnia, increases energy, and relieves chronic fatigue syndrome. Other claims for DHEA(S) are that it improves self-image, elevates mood, increases libido, and eliminates sexual dysfunction. DHEA(S) has also been said to retard aging and allow one to age gracefully with better stress management, a sharper mind, and an improved short-term memory. There are also unfounded claims for the impact of DHEA(S) on other disease processes, specifically that it lessens the effects of Alzheimer's disease, decreases cancer risks, decreases heart disease, improves the body's infection-fighting capability, and reduces arthralgia. Many readers will recognize that these are the same claims made for the male and female sex hormones, testosterone and estrogen.

A distinction must be made between media hype and actual scientific evidence. Experimental research with rabbits and mice indicate that DHEA seems to inhibit atherosclerosis (hardening of the arteries) and prolong life. Other probable benefits include increased libido and an elevated sense of well-being.

Some interesting, but not very useful, research findings suggest that both smoking and moderate use of alcohol (defined as two drinks per day) increases the body's level of DHEA(S). In men, weight loss also seems to increase DHEA. One study shows that higher levels of DHEA decrease the risk of heart attacks. In women, it also appears that estrogen replacement decreases the level of DHEA(S).

The current status of DHEA was reviewed in the October 11, 1996, issue of the *Medical Letter*. In the opening paragraph, the article notes that DHEA is being marketed as a "food supplement" in health food stores. It has *not*, however, been approved for *any* indication by the U.S. Food and Drug Administration (FDA). In one study, fifty milligrams/day of DHEA were given to thirteen men and seventeen women aged forty to seventy. The blood levels of DHEA in these subjects were found to be similar to those of young adults. The subjects reported an increase in physical and psychological well-being. Another study using 100 milligrams/day produced similar results. It was unclear whether DHEA had any effect on body composition or fat distribution.

The *Medical Letter* reports that there have also been some other interesting research findings on the relationship of DHEA to other health conditions. Plasma levels of DHEA in men (but not women) over the age of fifty were found to be inversely related to death from cardiovascular disease. DHEA has also been associated in a reduction of viral load in HIV-infected patients with AIDS. Another study reported that 200 milligrams/day of DHEA given for three months improved systemic lupus.

The adverse side effects reported by subjects who took DHEA in these studies were androgenic (masculinizing) in nature. In women, these side effects included acne, hair loss, hirsutism (male pattern of hair), and deepening of the voice. It is important to note that hirsutism and voice changes may be irreversible. In men, DHEA can stimulate the growth of prostate cancer (just as estrogen can stimulate the growth of breast cancer and endometrial cancer in women). The effect of DHEA on growth of breast and endometrial cancers is unknown.

The summary section of the *Medical Letter* article states, "There is no convincing evidence DHEA has any beneficial effect on aging or any disease. Patients would be well advised not to take it." The conclusion of this article should be taken seriously, as more physicians read the *Medical Letter* than any other medical report. Because of the high stature of its editors, contributing editors, and editorial advisory board, it has the universal respect of the medical world.

DHEA and DHEA(S) as "Dietary Supplements"

DHEA has been recently commanding a lot of media attention with attributions of almost miraculous youthening and health-enhancing powers. Some of the claims made for the benefits of DHEA and DHEA(S) have arisen from scientific studies. Unfortunately, most of the popularity and the hype for these hormones are built on the placebo effect. The placebo effect refers to the expectations a person has that they will benefit from a using a substance or product.

For the time being, the use of DHEA should be avoided because there is no convincing scientific evidence for its use. Large doses of DHEA should especially be avoided as the side effects from large doses (taken orally) are suspected to be the same as for overdoses of testosterone (prostate enlargement, increased rate of growth of prostate cancer, and liver disease). It is possible that taking DHEA may also increase the risk of developing prostate cancer. Overdosing on DHEA has essentially the same effects as overdosing on anabolic steroids.

At the present time, DHEA is in the same uncertain position as many other "magical" drugs in the market today that are being promoted as nutritional or dietary supplements. Because of the demand by consumers and inspired by premature publicity from studies and the profit motive, there is widespread unethical and potentially harmful use of DHEA.

Because of a loophole in federal law, any substance can be sold without a prescription over the counter by designating it a "dietary supplement" (unless previously designated otherwise by the FDA). Many chemicals, both natural and synthetic, are sold as dietary supplements although it is abundantly clear that they are not. Unfortunately, DHEA is yet another example of this problem.

No laws protect consumers from products labeled as dietary supplements. These fall outside the FDA's jurisdiction so there is absolutely no control over the raw materials used in their production or processing. There is also no requirement for concentration, potency, packaging standards, or product review. To offer an extreme example, horse manure could be ground up, colored, put in capsules, labeled as a dietary supplement, and sold as a cure for heart disease, cancer, diabetes, or whatever is of current concern to consumers.

The Placebo Effect

The reason that questionable or even harmful products labeled as "dietary supplements" survive, and even thrive, in the marketplace is because of their *placebo effect*. The placebo effect is a physical or emotional change occurring after a substance is taken that is not the result of the substance itself. Instead, the change is due to the person's expectations of receiving benefit from the substance. Like stress, the placebo effect is very real and can affect both the mind and body. Anyone can be vulnerable to the placebo effect regardless of their intelligence or educational level.

The strength of the placebo effect relates to a number of factors such as the amount of hype, the cost of the product, or the amount of discomfort experienced when using the product. To put it simply, the greater the hype, the stronger the placebo effect. The higher the price, or the more inconvenient and uncomfortable the product is (e.g., an injection versus an oral medication), the stronger the placebo effect. The more foreign the setting of treatment, the stronger the placebo effect (e.g., cancer treatments in Mexico). The more outlandish the product, the stronger the placebo effect (e.g., green slime from stagnant lakes). The greater the promotion celebration, the stronger the placebo effect (advertising campaigns make use of this phenomenon extensively). The more prestigious the advocate or spokesperson, the stronger the placebo effect (e.g., a TV celebrity versus the local pharmacist).

One other factor helps explain the power of the placebo effect. People who enthusiastically accepted a therapy or treatment and then later found out it was ineffective or harmful don't want to admit to having made a mistake. After all, no one likes being a "sucker." Most people are very reluctant to admit their foolish decisions to either themselves or others. Even the truth can't always counteract the power of the placebo effect. Anecdotal reports, testimonies from friends, and reports by medical professionals or responsible journalists can be meaningless in the face of the placebo effect. Thus, the quackery goes on uninhibited.

Anabolic Steroids

Steroid is a generic term that is often misused. Steroids are a large group of naturally occurring organic compounds that includes cholesterol, bile products, adrenal hormones, and sex hormones. There are numerous types of steroids such as anabolic steroids, sex steroids, and adrenal steroids. Cortisone and its many derivatives are adrenal steroids.

Anabolic steroids were first synthesized in the 1930s but were not publicized until after World War II when they were used to restore body weight in concentration camp survivors.

The anabolic steroids are synthetic male sex hormones derived from, and chemically similar to, testosterone and with similar effects on the body. *Anabolic* means that the steroid has the characteristic of increasing constructive metabolism such as building new muscle tissue.

Testosterone and the other anabolic steroids are very similar chemically and biologically; the arrangement of the atoms is approximately the same with just one carbon atom difference. For example, the steroid Deniable has the same chemical structure as testosterone except for the addition of a group with one carbon atom and three hydrogen atoms. A fundamental rule of pharmacology is that similar chemicals have similar biological effects on the body. They both affect the same receptors in the body, so the body responses to the two are also almost identical. But researchers have difficulty comparing the effects of testosterone and the anabolic steroids on muscle development and performance because of the extreme disparity in doses. The standard dose for anabolic steroids is hundreds of times that for testosterone. Theoretically, testosterone could also be administered in very large doses to achieve the same body-building results as anabolic steroids, but the actual differences in the effects on the human body are unknown at this time.

Like testosterone, anabolic steroids affect the bone marrow, increase the circulation of red blood cells, and have been used to correct certain types of anemia. They have also shown to be of benefit when used to treat a condition called hereditary angioneurotic edema (excessive fluid in a certain location) probably due to their effects on the liver. Recent research indicates that sex steroid–thyroid hormone mixtures might be useful in treating skin pigmentation disorders such as vitiligo.

Proteins and the
Use of Amino Acid Supplements

The body needs protein to sustain and increase muscle mass. Adequate protein intake is also needed for healthy bones because the matrix containing calcium compounds is composed mostly of protein material.

Proteins are complex chemicals composed of carbon, hydrogen, oxygen, and nitrogen; some also contain sulfur. The presence of nitrogen is the most distinguishing characteristic. Proteins are the principal constituents of the protoplasm of all cells.

Proteins are composed of amino acids. There are twenty different amino acids in proteins. Nine of these are classified as essential amino acids, which means that the body cannot synthesize them so they must be ingested from sources outside the body. Americans get most of their proteins from animal food sources, but there are excellent plant sources of protein foods as well.

Many amino acid preparations are promoted for various purposes, especially to athletes and body builders. They are a concentrated source but not superior to other sources. The same amino acids are found in meat, poultry, eggs, milk, legumes, and other plant sources.

The Effects of Aging on the Body

Atherosclerosis

The most pronounced cause of many of the symptoms associated with aging is the decreased flow of blood in the arteries. With time, the internal dimensions of the arteries decrease, which reduces the blood supply to all the organs and tissues. The reduction in oxygen carried by the blood reduces the activity and metabolism in the cells; they become less efficient.

The internal dimensions of blood vessels decrease naturally because of atherosclerosis. In atherosclerosis, the inner walls of the arteries are thickened by deposits of lipid (fatty) materials followed by the production of fibrous tissue in a process called *fibrosis*, which is somewhat similar to scar formation. The blood vessels lose their elasticity and become less compliant to internal pressures. A generation ago, this process was poorly understood and called "hardening of the arteries." This used to be noted on death certificates as "dying of old age."

There is a great variation in the rate of progression of atherosclerosis among individuals. It progresses more quickly in men than in women. Other factors that accelerate the process are unfavorable hereditary patterns, hyperlipidemia, especially excess low-density lipoprotein (LDL, or "bad" cholesterol), hypertension, diabetes, obesity, and tobacco smoking. Interest has arisen in recent years about whether stress might also be a factor. It may be that Type-A personalities are also more susceptible.

In addition to heart and brain vessels, the peripheral vessels in the arms and legs are susceptible to the changes associated with atherosclerosis. In the leg muscles, less oxygen decreases strength and endurance and, in advanced stages, causes pain. The peripheral arteries that supply blood to the penis are also affected. In the penis, when there is impaired blood supply, less blood is available to create an erection. Less blood flow means less oxygen to the tissues they supply. When less oxygen is supplied to tissues, their function is impeded. An inadequate supply of oxygen to the heart muscles (supplied by the coronary arteries) causes fatigue and impaired endurance. It is also one cause of heart failure. In the brain, the thought processes are slowed.

The rate of change is not the same for all parts of the body and varies from one person to another. The body's organ systems have considerable reserve capacity, so the reduction in function is not apparent until late in the chronological life of an individual. Each organ system's function declines at a different physiological rate. The slowdown is more apparent in some tissues than in others. In the skin, for example, the blood supply affects the amount of collagen, which provides the elasticity in the skin. The reduced blood flow decreases the amount of collagen and leads to wrinkling. This is especially noticeable in those who have smoked cigarettes for many years because nicotine constricts the small arteries of the skin even further.

Some conditions accelerate the progress of atherosclerosis. The most commonly recognized is the thickening of the artery lining by cholesterol plaques. Cholesterol itself is actually only one of the lipids involved, but high cholesterol is one of the main causes. The lining of arteries is called *endothelium,* and it's under this lining and in the adjacent walls that the lipids accumulate, thickening the walls and reducing the internal diameter. In the past, the process of atherosclerosis—including plaque formation—was believed to be irreversible, but more recently most cardiologists and other clinicians believe the process can be reversed. This is accomplished by reducing the lipids in the bloodstream, especially the LDL ("bad" cholesterol), so fewer lipids are available to accumulate. For those at high risk (for example those with coronary heart disease) the goal is to bring the LDL below the reference and normal range, to less than 100 milligrams per deciliter of blood.

Other Conditions

In addition to atherosclerosis, a few other "natural" changes are associated with aging. The abrupt atrophy of women's ovaries, as occurs in menopause, and the gradual decrease in male testicular function are both universal. Male pattern baldness is also considered a normal aging process, resulting from the hair follicles dying.

Another natural but reversible condition that accelerates aging is hypothyroidism, that is, inadequate amounts of thyroid hormones made by the thyroid gland. There are no immediate symptoms of hypothyroidism; the aging changes are gradual like the slow aging changes of the skin. The related aging effects on various parts of the body are essentially the same as those of decreased blood supply. The symptoms that may bring hypothyroidism to the attention of the individual or physician are weakness, fatigue, lethargy, dry and/or coarse skin, swelling of extremities, cold intolerance, decreased sweating, huskiness of the voice, slight weight gain in the presence of a reduced appetite, impaired memory, constipation, and muscle cramps. Hypothyroidism is easily, quickly, and accurately diagnosed with a blood test of the thyroid-stimulating hormone (TSH). Hypothyroidism is most often a natural event of aging as demonstrated by its higher frequency in older people, but it can also result from a virus or bacterial infection involving the thyroid gland. It is effectively treated with oral thyroid replacement with an inexpensive prescription medication.

The role of environmental factors on aging are, as yet, not well understood, although solid evidence indicates that some environmental substances cause or accelerate certain diseases. One example that has received a lot of publicity is the effect of second-hand cigarette smoke on the development of lung cancer and chronic obstructive pulmonary disease (COPD). Another example is exposure to asbestos. However, causing disease is one thing and accelerating the aging process is another.

Psychological disturbances can cause a number of physical abnormalities, like headaches or indigestion. But here again, causing or accelerating disease is not the same as aging. Despite the popularity of the myth, worry and anxiety do not cause gray hair.

Medical Conditions Impacting Testosterone

Among the rare conditions that affect testosterone circulation are some genetic defects and developmental conditions affecting various glands of the endocrine system including the testes, adrenals, and thyroid.

Klinefelter's syndrome is the most common cause of primary testicular failure, resulting in impairment of both spermatogenesis (sperm formation) and testosterone production. The fundamental defect that identifies Klinefelter's is the presence of one or more extra X chromosomes. Klinefelter's is not usually detected until puberty and is characterized by small, firm testes, azoospermia (absence of sperm in the semen), gynecomastia (enlarged breasts), and testosterone levels in the low or low-normal range. The condition affects one in every 400 to 500 men.

Noonan's, also called male *Turner's syndrome,* can occur sporadically but is often hereditary. Characteristics of this syndrome are short stature, ptosis (drooping of the upper eyelid), low-set ears, small jaws, webbed neck, mental retardation, and impairment of both spermatogenesis and testosterone production. With this condition, fertility is variable and testosterone levels fall to the low or low-normal range.

If testosterone is not present during the three to fourteen weeks of gestation, there will be ambiguity in the development of the external male genitalia in the fetus, a condition called *pseudohermaphroditism.* This condition does not allow the normal enlargement of the penis or scrotum at puberty. The prostate and seminal vesicles, necessary to produce an ejaculate (semen), do not develop. In addition, there is an absence of the male pattern of hair growth, the voice box fails to mature, and the development of muscles and bone growth is disrupted.

Another developmental disorder, *cryptorchidism,* prevents one or both testes from descending from the lower abdomen, where they start in life, to the scrotum during puberty.

Normally, the testes begin this descent into the scrotum during the eighth month of fetal life. The disorder occurs in 3 to 4 percent of newborn males, but in most cases the testes do descend during the first year of life, so by age one only 0.5 percent of boys still demonstrate the disorder. If a testis remains in the abdomen beyond puberty, it loses its ability to produce sperm, so if the condition affects both gonads, the man is sterile. The unilateral condition (only one testis does not descend) is five to ten times more common than the bilateral. Cryptorchidism does not usually interfere with testosterone production because the Leydig cells usually remain intact. Surgical correction of the defect is advisable before puberty to preserve fertility and prevent the likelihood of cancer. An undescended testis is twenty to thirty times more likely to undergo malignant changes than those located in the scrotum. Since this condition is surgically treatable, it is an extremely rare cause of testosterone deficiency.

If an adolescent boy contracts a case of mumps that "go down," that is, if the virus spreads to his gonads, his testosterone production may be permanently impaired, but only if the virus infects both gonads. If one testis is missing or has impaired function, the remaining healthy testis is fully capable of producing an adequate number of sperm to fertilize a woman's egg. The total count may be moderately lower, but the number is more than adequate to produce conception. The healthy remaining testis is also fully capable of producing an adequate amount of testosterone.

Generalized debilitating diseases such as advanced cancers, advanced lung diseases such as chronic pulmonary obstructive disease, heart failure, and other cardiovascular diseases, advanced liver disease such as cirrhosis, and severe malnutrition can also reduce testosterone output. These diseases and conditions impair the body's ability to supply the nutritional needs of all the tissues, including those of the gonads. Testosterone deficiency is considered an indirect effect of these diseases. The inadequately supplied tissues either reduce their functional output or die and are not replaced.

Hyperprolactinemia, too much of the hormone prolactin, exists in an estimated 25 percent of all infertile women, but it is much less common in men. Prolactin is a hormone produced by the anterior pituitary gland in both men and women. In women it stimulates lactation in the postpartum period. It does not play a role in the regulation of male gonadal function, but when an excess is produced, it leads to *hypogonadism,* or testosterone deficiency. The upper normal range for prolactin in the blood of men is fifteen to twenty nanograms/deciliter. In addition, some medications may increase the production of the hormone including tricyclic antidepressants, antipsychotics (the phenothiazines), and antihypertension agents.

Tumors of the pituitary gland can affect testosterone production. A benign tumor, or *adenoma,* of the anterior pituitary may cause prolactin production in excessive amounts. When the tumor is present, the blood level of prolactin will exceed 200 milligrams/milliliter. When the tumors are small, the condition can be treated medically with bromocriptin (Parlodel) or other medications. Medicinal treatment is less reliable for treating the larger tumors, and surgical intervention is often used if there is obstruction to the flow of cerebrospinal fluid or if the tumor is unresponsive to medical therapy. Many physicians will order a prolactin blood test when a testosterone test shows a low hormone level to rule out hyperprolactinemia as a cause. Five percent or more cases of low testosterone levels are caused by hyperprolactinemia. When prolactin is high, men typically have low libido and some degree of impotence. Fortunately, treatment of this condition has a very high success rate.

Benign and malignant tumors of the testes, adrenals, and thyroid glands can begin in childhood or adulthood and can affect testosterone production. Any cancer that involves both testes to the degree that the testosterone cells (the Leydig cells) are completely replaced by the cancer eliminates testosterone production. Unfortunately, radiation and chemotherapy treatments for any type of cancer also affect testosterone production. Both radiation and chemotherapy can destroy the Leydig cells along with the cancer cells. These are irreversible changes, so the patient and his partner should be informed of this consequence before therapy is started.

Castration

Castration (complete removal or "closure of the testes") abruptly reduces the body's testosterone level, since the testes produce 95 percent of a man's testosterone.

Erection may occur in the absence of testosterone, but the frequency is less and there is usually less firmness. Boys before puberty, while producing very little testosterone, have frequent erections; even newborn babies have them. Castrated animals, such as stallions, continue to have sizable erections.

Castration is performed occasionally for the treatment of certain advanced cancers. It does not totally prevent the body's testosterone production capacity but is definitely sufficient to slow down the progression of prostate cancer.

Sexual response to castration is variable. In general, the least change is seen in young, highly sexual males. But all castrated males have a marked lowering of their testosterone level that is accompanied by a fall in their libido. With less active thoughts of sex, a man has less need for sexual gratification. This may be a greater problem to his partner than to himself, but most loving men are able to satisfy their mates' needs for sexual gratification. Many of the men with advanced prostate cancer are older and less active sexually and do not see this as a major problem.

Postoperatively, most castrated men seem discontented. This is a natural consequence of removing the testosterone that has maintained their sense of well-being. But the degree of mood change is difficult to assess because a man who knows he has a progressing cancer is certain to be somewhat dysphoric. In men who have had little or no preoperative experience with impotence, most continue to have satisfactory erections, but the usual pattern is a gradual decrease in erectile powers. Orgasmic function usually parallels the changes in libido and potency.

"Chemical castration" is now in the news quite often. Technically, it is not castration at all since the gonads aren't touched, but rather it is the reduction of testosterone levels by the administration of testosterone-reducing drugs such as Depo Provera. Chemical castration is used primarily, by court order, to reduce the sex drive of sex offenders, usually pedophiles. The effects dissipate almost immediately when the weekly injections of the medication are withdrawn. It is not a particularly effective treatment for sex offenders because it only reduces the libido—it doesn't eliminate it—and it doesn't curtail a man's ability to have an erection or to ejaculate. Many sex offenders are motivated by violent urges rather than sexual ones, and the violence is not due to a surplus of testosterone but rather to disturbing psychological factors.

Comparing Deficiencies:
Testosterone in Men and Estrogen in Women

Testosterone deficiency and estrogen deficiency both refer to an inadequate level of circulating sex hormone in the bloodstream. Other than the obvious difference—one being a condition in men and the other in women—there are additional differences. However, there are also significant similarities in testosterone and estrogen deficiencies.

The underlying causes of estrogen and testosterone deficiencies are the same: gonadal failure. Except in rare cases, the failures are irreversible in both men and women. Medical science has not, as yet, successfully transplanted either ovaries or testes.

The primary information source for diagnosing sex hormone deficiency in women is the medical history, whereas for men it is the laboratory test results. In diagnosing testosterone deficiency, the clinician uses the history of symptoms and prior illness or injuries that affected the testes. Unlike estrogen deficiency diagnosis, a man's family history is of little, if any, value. The only significant part of the physical examination that is of use in determining the diagnosis is that of the scrotal contents. Laboratory tests are an extremely important part of the diagnosis process, whereas testing a woman's blood does not add much in the assessment of estrogen deficiency.

The chemical structure of estrogen and testosterone are quite similar; thus, some of their effects are similar. For example, both retard the loss of minerals from the bones that leads to fractures. The differences in chemical structure are responsible for differences in male and female response when there is a deficiency in testosterone or estrogen.

Estrogen deficiency, in the form of menopause, occurs in all women, but testosterone deficiency does not develop in all men. The ages of onset are similar, but the physical changes are different. Treatment for both deficiencies is replacement. Much more scientific research has been done on female hormonal deficiency than on the male condition, but the gap is beginning to close. Results of the research have led to improvements and more choices, like skin patches, in the route of administration of sex hormones.

Normal aging changes in the gonads are most often responsible for both testosterone and estrogen deficiencies, but the process is much more abrupt in women than in men. Except in the very rare cases of injury or severe disease of the gonads, the onset of testosterone deficiency is extremely gradual. The drop in testosterone in men in their thirties and forties is almost imperceptible symptomatically or by laboratory testing. Only as the slow decline in testosterone continues into the late fifties and early sixties can it be confirmed by lab tests. There are no reliable statistics on what percentage of men become testosterone deficient at certain ages—for example, what percentage of men seek medical attention in their sixties for symptoms due to the deficiency. Recent medical studies suggest this number is higher than believed a few years ago. Educated estimates now run as high as 60 percent ascribing sexual dysfunction to testosterone deficiency.

Estrogen deficiency is most often associated with the normal onset of menopause in women. One hundred percent of women become estrogen deficient at some time in their lives; however, the severity of the related menopause syndrome varies greatly, as does the age of onset. The onset of menopause is most commonly in the fifties but can occur as early as a woman's late thirties.

The terms *menopause, estrogen deficiency, climacteric,* and *change of life* are often used interchangeably. Estrogen deficiency refers to a low level of circulating female hormones in a woman's body, whereas the other three terms usually refer to a syndrome. This syndrome includes symptoms as well as physical and chemical changes. There are no comparable terms in popular usage for the changes men experience. Occasionally the lay and professional medical literature refer to *testosterone deficiency* and *male menopause.* (These terms are not synonymous, as revealed in Chapter 8.)

Symptoms occurring in estrogen deficiency vary widely, and this variation is only somewhat related to the degree of estrogen decline, whereas the degree of drop in testosterone in males is quite clearly related to the nature and severity of the symptoms. The symptoms of testosterone deficiency are more specific and limited than those of estrogen deficiency. In both conditions the deficiencies detract from good health. They both reduce the feeling of well-being and vigor. Inadequate sex hormones contribute to osteoporosis in men and women, and sexual dysfunction can ensue when there is a deficiency of either hormone (see Table A-1).

Significant differences in the prognosis for men and women are evident when they develop deficiencies in their sex hormones, but the prognosis is quite similar between the two with replacement therapy. There is not general agreement in the medical community whether estrogen is needed for women in their eighties and beyond or at what age it can be discontinued. Nor do physicians agree on the best doses of estrogen to be used during these advanced years.

Both men and women suffer the mental and physical changes of decreasing sex hormone production by their bodies. The symptoms are somewhat dissimilar, but untreated the prognosis is similarly unfavorable. Both men and women have an improved prognosis with hormone replacement.

Table A-1.   Male and Female Sex Hormone Deficiencies

	Men	Women
Age at onset	55	45–55
Duration of decline	Remainder of life	5–10 years
Nature of decline	Very gradual	Abrupt
Primary gland	Testes	Ovaries
Controlling gland	Pituitary	
Organs or tissues affected	Muscle, bone, genitalia	Bladder, vagina, blood vessels, heart
Effect on reproduction	Variable (decreased)	Sterile
Diagnosis	Physical exam	Laboratory tests
Blood tests	Testosterone	FSH*
Physical changes	Muscle weakness, sexual dysfunction	Vaginal lining atrophy, hot flashes
Psychological changes	Apathy, reduced libido	Anxiety, depression
Treatment	Testosterone replacement	Estrogen replacement
Adjunctive treatment	Restore physical health	
	Healthy lifestyle	
Duration of replacement	Usually lifetime	
Dosage	Adequate to control	

* Follicle Stimulating Hormone of the pituitary

SUGGESTED READING

Bahr, Robert. 1992. *The Virility Factors*. Mobile, AL: Factor
Press.

Bennett, Alan H. 1994. *Impotence: Diagnosis and Management of
Erectile Dysfunction*. Philadelphia: Saunders.

Gilbaugh, James H. 1989. *A Doctor's Guide to Men's Private Parts*.
New York: Crown.

Hill, Aubrey M. 1993. *Viropause/Andropause: The Male
Menopause*. Far Hills, NJ: New Horizon Press.

Masters, William M., and Virginia E. Johnson. 1970/1980.
Human Sexual Inadequacy. Boston: Little, Brown; New
York: Bantam.

Rako, Susan. 1996. *The Hormone of Desire*. New York: Harmony
Books.

Regelson, William. 1996. *The Superhormone Promise*. New York:
Simon and Schuster.

Sahelian, Roy. 1996. *DHEA: A Practical Guide*. Garden City, New
York: Avery.

GLOSSARY

adenoma—a benign tumor of glandular origin.

adrenal cortex—the outer layer of the gland that secretes steroid hormones.

adrenal glands—two anatomical structures located above both kidneys.

adrenal medulla—the central portion of the adrenals that secrete adrenaline and related chemicals.

aerobic—occurring in the presence of oxygen.

aerobics—a system of physical conditioning to improve respiratory and circulatory function.

albumin—water-soluble proteins occurring in blood and muscle.

Alzheimer's disease—a progressive degenerative disease of the brain.

amino acid—chemicals containing nitrogen and hydrogen; chief components of protein.

anabolic—refers to the constructive part of metabolism by which energy is made available to the body.

androgen—any substance that is conducive to masculinization.

androgenic—producing masculine characteristics.

andropause—male menopause; a medically defined psychological condition of dysphoria or unease that occurs in men between the ages of forty and sixty.

androstenediol/androstenedione—androgens that are produced in the body's process of making other hormones (e.g., testosterone).

anemia—a condition in which the body is deficient in red blood cells and/or their components.

angina—pain, now almost exclusively used to denote angina pectoris (pain of the chest).

angiotensin-converting enzyme inhibitors (ACE inhibitors)—a newer group of medications used for treating high blood pressure.

anorgasmia—failure to experience orgasm in coitus.

antioxidant—a substance that prevents or retards deterioration by the action of oxygen.

aphrodisiac—exciting the libido.

arrhenoblastoma—a growth of the ovary, sometimes causing defeminization and virilization.

atherosclerosis—a very common condition in which plaques containing cholesterol are formed in the lining of arteries.

arthralgia—pain of the body joints.

arthritis—inflammation of the body joints.

axon—that part of a nerve cell by which impulses move away from the cell body.

azoospermia—absence of sperm in the semen.

benign prostatic hyperplasia (BPH)—non-malignant enlargement of the prostate (gland).

beta blockers—one group of drugs used for treating high blood pressure. Abbreviated term for beta-adrenoceptor blocker.

buccal—pertaining to, or directed toward, the cheek.

carcinoma—a malignant new growth made up of certain (epithelial) cells that tend to infiltrate surrounding tissue.

cardiovascular—relating to the heart and blood vessels.

castration—surgical removal of the testes or ovaries.

catabolism—destructive metabolism resulting in the breakdown of materials within the body.

central nervous system—brain and spinal cord.

chlamydia—a genus of bacteria that multiply only within a cell.

chromosome—a structure in the nucleus containing a thread of DNA, which transmits generic information.

chronic—persisting over a long period of time.

circadian—characterized by or occurring in approximately 24-hour periods or cycles.

cirrhosis—a liver disease characterized by loss of normal structure.

climacteric—a period in life, at the termination of the reproductive cycle, when endocrine, somatic, and psychic changes occur.

clitoris—a small, elongated, erectile body, situated at the upper end of the vulva of the female external genitalia, corresponding to the male penis.

cognition—the act or process by the mind of knowing; becoming aware through perception; aspects of perceiving, thinking, and remembering.

coitus—sexual intercourse achieved by insertion of a man's penis into a woman's vagina.

collagen—the protein substance of the white fibers of skin, tendon, bone, and cartilage.

congenital—existing at or before birth.

coronary—denotes arteries that supply the heart muscle.

Glossary

corpus cavernosum—distensible, spongy tissue of the penis.

cortex—outer layer (e.g. of the adrenal glands) that secretes certain chemicals.

corticosteroid—any of various adrenal cortex steroids, excluding sex hormones.

cortisone—one of the hormones secreted by the adrenal cortex.

cryptorchidism—a developmental defect characterized by failure of the testes to descend into the scrotum.

dehydroepiandrosterone—an androgenic hormone, synthesized from cholesterol, and occurring naturally in the body.

demineralization—the process of mineral loss, often used to describe the loss of calcium and phosphorus from the bones.

dendrite—the receptive servers of a nerve cell (neuron).

detumescence—diminution or subsidence of swelling or erection.

diagnostic—distinctive of a disease; a symptom serving as supporting evidence in a diagnosis.

diastolic blood pressure—the second and lower figure of a blood pressure determination occurring during the dilation phase of the heart beat.

dihydrotestosterone (DHT)—a powerful androgenic hormone produced from testosterone by the action of 5 alpha-reductase.

diurnal—occurring during the day.

dopamine—a chemical formed in the body that acts as a mediator in the central nervous system.

dyspareunia—difficult or painful intercourse.

dyspepsia—impairment of the function of digestion; upper abdominal discomfort following meals.

dysphoria—disquiet, restlessness, malaise, unpleasant mood.

edema—the presence of a large amount of fluid in the tissue spaces of the body.

ejaculate—to suddenly expel semen in the male orgasm.

ejaculation—the sudden expulsion of semen in male orgasm.

emission—a discharge; specifically an involuntary discharge of semen.

endocrine—secreting internally; applied to organs whose function is to secrete into the blood a substance (hormone) that has a specific effect on another organ.

endometriosis—a condition in which tissue resembling the uterus lining occurs aberrantly in various locations of the pelvic cavity.

endometrium—the inner lining of the uterus.

endothelium—a layer of cells lining the cavities of the heart, blood vessels, and certain cavities of the body.

epididymis—a cord-like structure behind the testes that provides for storage or transit of spermatozoa.

epiphysis—the end of long bones developed from a bone center beginning as a cartilage.

erection—the condition of being made rigid and elevated, as the penis when filled with blood.

ergot—a fungus that replaces the seed of a grass, such as rye, used medicinally for its contractile effect on certain muscles.

estradiol—the most potent, naturally occurring estrogen, from the ovaries.

estrogen—a female hormone formed in the ovary.

estrone—an estrogen produced by the body from estradiol.

etiochololanlone—a body chemical formed from testosterone and excreted in the urine.

etiology—the study of factors that cause disease; the cause(s) or origin of a disease or disorder.

fallopian tube—either of a pair of tubes conducting the egg from the ovary to the uterus.

fetus—a developing human from seven or eight weeks after conception; an unborn offspring.

fibrosis—the formation of fibrous tissue or fibrous degeneration.

5 alpha-reductase—a body enzyme that converts testosterone to a more active form, dihydrotestosterone.

follicle stimulating hormone (FSH)—a hormone secreted by the pituitary, which, when reaching the ovary via the bloodstream, causes the formation of a cystic structure containing the egg. In the male it stimulates the testes to produce sperm.

free radicals—commonly used to designate an extremely active oxygen atom that carries an unpaired electron.

gastrointestinal—pertaining to the stomach and the intestine.

genitourinary—pertaining to the internal and external organs of the genital system and the urinary system.

genitalia—the various internal and external organs concerned with reproduction.

gestation—the period of development of the unborn young from the time of fertilization of the egg until birth.

gland—an aggregation of cells that are specialized to secrete materials not related to their ordinary metabolic needs.

glans—the cap-shaped expansion of corpus at the end of the penis.

globulin—a class of proteins that are insoluble in water.

gonad—an organ that produces mature sperm (the male testis) or eggs (the female ovary).

gonadotropic—refers to hormones of the pituitary that influence the gonads.

gonorrhea orchitis—infection of the testes by the gonococcus bacteria.

gynecomastia—excessive development or enlargement of the male mammary glands.

half-life—as pertains to drugs, indicates the time when half of the drug remains active.

hematocrit—the volume of packed red blood cells in a given blood specimen.

hemoglobin—the oxygen carrying pigment of red blood cells formed in the bone marrow.

hemorrhagic—pertaining to hemorrhage or tissue into which hemorrhage has occurred.

hereditary angioedema—collection of body fluids in tissue, especially the lips and other areas of the face, transmitted as an autosomal dominant trait.

high-density lipoprotein (HDL)—a very large molecule found in the blood, part of which is cholesterol; "protects" the arteries from the undesirable effect of cholesterol; the "good" cholesterol.

hippocampus—a part of the brain.

hirsutism—abnormal hairiness, especially an adult male pattern of hair distribution in women.

hormone—a chemical substance, produced in the body by an organ or cells of an organ, which has a specific regulatory or stimulatory effect on the activity of another organ.

hydrocodone—a synthetic product with analgesic effects similar to codeine, but more active than codeine.

hyperlipidemia—a general term for elevated concentration of any or all of the lipids in the blood, such as cholesterol.

hyperprolactinemia—increased level of prolactin in the blood.

hypertension—high blood pressure.

hyperthyroidism—excess secretion of thyroid hormones.

hysterectomy—surgical removal of the uterus.

impotence—lack of power, chiefly of copulative power in the male; incapable of sexual intercourse.

insulin—a protein hormone secreted by certain cells of the pancreas; exogenous insulin is used for control of diabetes.

insulin dependent diabetes mellitis (Type I), (IDDM)—a type of diabetes in which circulating insulin is virtually absent.

intercourse—coitus; sexual joining of male and female.

intramuscular—within the substance of the muscle.

introitus—a general term for the entrance to a cavity, as the entrance to the vagina.

intromission—insertion of the penis into the vagina.

jaundice—a syndrome characterized by deposition of bile pigment into the skin, resulting in a yellow appearance.

Klinefelter's syndrome—a condition characterized by small testes and variable decrease of masculinization and infertility.

lactation—the secretion of milk.

larynx—the voice box.

Leydig cells—clusters of cells constituting the hormonal tissue of the testes, which produce androgens, chiefly testosterone; also called interstitial cells.

limbic system—a term loosely applied to a group of brain structures; important in aspects of emotion and behavior.

lipid—any of a heterogeneous group of fats that are water soluble; in the body they serve as a source of fuel and are important constituents of cell structure.

low-density lipoprotein (LDL)—a smaller lipid molecule contained in compounds; the "bad" cholesterol.

Glossary

luteinizing hormone—a hormone of the pituitary that instigates and maintains the second portion of the menstrual cycle; in the male it stimulates the development and functional activity of the Leydig cells.

lymphatic system—the vessels and nodes that transport a clear fluid from body tissues to the blood vessels.

male menopause—layman's term for andropause.

malignant—tending to become progressively worse and resulting in death; having the properties of invasion and metastasis.

masturbation—self-stimulation of the genitals for sexual pleasure.

melatonin—a hormone synthesized by the pineal body of the brain whose activity is influenced by exposure to light.

menarche—the establishment or beginning of menstrual function.

menopause—cessation of menstruation in the human female; climacteric.

menses—the monthly flow of blood from the genital tract of women.

menstrual—pertaining to menses.

metabolism—the sum of all physical and chemical processes by which living organized substance is produced and maintained; also the transformation by which energy is made available for use by the body.

metabolite—any substance produced by metabolism.

metastasis—the transfer of disease from one organ or part to another not directly connected to it.

methyltestosterone—a synthetic androgen derived from cholesterol, having action similar to testosterone; used in replacement therapy.

mucous membrane—the sheet of cells of lining tissues or organs that produce slime or moisture.

myocardial infarction—heart muscle tissue death due to deprived blood supply by obstruction of an artery by a thrombus (clot).

neuralgia—a paroxysmal pain that extends along the course of a nerve.

neuritis—inflammation of a nerve.

neurological—pertaining to the nerves; the medical science that deals with the nervous system.

neurons—any of the conducting cells of the nervous system.

neurotransmitters—a group of substances, including adrenaline, dopamine, and serotonin, that are released on excitation from the axon of the nervous system to excite or inhibit the target cell.

nitric oxide—a compound consisting of nitrogen and oxygen, which paralyzes and relaxes the muscles of the blood vessels (e.g. in the penis) so the muscles can expand in width.

non-insulin dependent diabetes (Type II), (NIDD)—a type of diabetes mellitus usually characterized by gradual onset and not requiring exogenous insulin for control.

Noonan's syndrome—a congenital complex of webbed neck, drooping of the upper eyelids, hypogonadism, and short stature.

orgasm—the climax of sexual excitement marked normally by ejaculation of semen by the male and by the release of tumescence in erectile organs of both sexes.

osteoporosis—abnormal loss of bone tissue; seen most commonly in the elderly.

ovary—sexual gland in which the ova (eggs) are formed.

ovulation—the production or discharge of an egg from the ovary in women.

ovum—the female reproductive cell; an egg.

oxidation—an increase of positive charges in an atom or ion of
a negative charge; biologically accomplished by removal
of a pair of hydrogen atoms from a molecule.

parathyroid glands—small tissues behind the thyroid gland
that secrete a substance that partially controls calcium
and phosphorous metabolism.

pharmacology—the science that deals with the origin, nature,
chemistry, effects, and uses of drugs.

phenothiazine—a group of psychotherapeutic agents that have
potent effects on the central nervous system with
hypnotic, antihistamine, and antivomiting effects.

placebo—a dummy medical treatment, having no
pharmacological activity against a patient's illness or
complaint; given for the psychophysiological effects.

plaque—a patch or flat area.

plasma—the fluid portion of the blood in which the
particulate components are suspended.

porphyria—a disturbance of the metabolism of porphyrin, a
compound found in the body, which can result in a
variety of conditions.

post-partum—after giving birth to a child.

posterior pituitary—a gland of the brain that secretes a
number of hormones into the bloodstream.

precursor—something that precedes; in biological processes,
a substance from which another is formed.

presenting symptoms—complaints patients make to the
physician at the first encounter.

priapism—abnormal erection of the penis, usually without
sexual desire and accompanied by pain.

progesterone—hormone produced by the corpus luteum after
ovulation in women.

progestin—the name given to progesterone-related agents.

prognosis—a forecast as to the probable outcome of a disease; the prospects of recovery as indicated by the symptoms and nature of the case.

prolactin—hormone secreted by the anterior pituitary that stimulates milk production in the breasts.

prostate—a gland in the male that surrounds the neck of the bladder and the upper urethra; the prostate contributes to the semen fluid.

prostate-specific antigen (PSA)—a chemical produced and secreted into the bloodstream by the prostate.

prostatectomy—surgical removal of the prostate.

prostatitis—inflammation of the prostate.

Prozac—the first of the serotonin-selective inhibitors used for depression.

pseudohermaphroditism—a condition in which the gonads are of one sex, but contradictions exist in the morphologic (form and structure) criteria of sex.

psychogenic—having symptoms of an emotional or psychological origin as opposed to having a physiological or organic basis.

psychosomatic—pertaining to the mind/body relationship; having bodily symptoms of psychic, emotional, or mental origins.

ptosis—a drooping of the upper eyelid.

puberty—the period during which the secondary sex characteristics begin to develop and the capacity of sexual reproduction is attained.

resorption—the loss of substance.

saccharide—one of a series of carbohydrates, including sugars.

scrotum—the pouch that contains the testes.

sebaceous glands—the glands of the skin that secrete an oily substance.

semen—the thick, whitish secretion of the reproductive organs in the male, composed of sperm and secretions from the prostate, seminal vesicles, and various other glands.

seminal vesicles—pouches attached to the back of the urinary bladder.

seminiferous tubules—channels in which the spermatozoa develop.

serotonin—a chemical synthesized by certain body cells, in neurons (nerve cells) and other tissues, which serves as a neurotransmitter and is a precursor to melatonin.

sertoli cells—cells of the testes that supply support and protection to the immature spermatozoa.

sperm—the cell of male reproduction; spermatozoa.

spermatogenesis—producing spermatozoa.

steroid—a group name for certain lipids, which includes progesterone, the sex hormones, and some of the adrenal hormones.

subcutaneous—beneath the skin.

sublingual—under the tongue.

substrate—a substance upon which an enzyme acts.

suspensory ligament—fibrous structure extending from the pubic bone to the penis that holds the penis in an elevated position during erection.

synapse—the site of functional apposition between neurons; where an impulse is transmitted from one neuron to another by either chemical or electrical means.

terminal hair—the coarse hair growing on various areas of the body during adult years.

testes—plural of testis; the male gonads normally situated in the scrotum.

testosterone—the hormone produced by certain cells of the testes that functions in the induction and maintenance of male secondary characteristics.

therapeutic trial—administration of a therapeutic substance and determination of its efficacy from the effects of the substance.

thrombosis—the formation, development, or presence of a thrombus (an aggregation of blood factors with entrapment of cells) causing vessel obstruction.

thymus—organs of the lymphatic system situated in the upper chest.

thyroid—a gland, situated in the lower part of the front of the neck, which secretes a hormone that plays a major role in regulating the metabolic rate of other tissues of the body.

thyroid stimulating hormone (TSH)—a hormone secreted by the pituitary gland that regulates the function of the thyroid gland.

thyrotoxicosis—an illness resulting from overactivity by the thyroid gland with multiple physical and psychological symptoms.

transurethral resection of the prostate (TURP)—surgical removal of obstructing prostate tissue by way of the urethra.

tricyclic antidepressives—a group of medications for treatment of depression, each of which have three cyclic configurations in the chemical structure.

triglyceride—a compound, found in the blood, consisting of three molecules of fatty acid.

TRT—testosterone replacement therapy.

Turner syndrome—a defect or absence of the secondary sex hormone resulting in variable abnormalities including joint deformities, cardiac condition, and webbing of the neck.

urethra—the canal conveying urine from the bladder to the exterior of the body.

urinalysis—a laboratory test of the urine.

uterus—the hollow muscular organ in females in which the fertilized egg becomes embedded and in which the embryo and fetus are nourished.

vagina—the canal in a female, extending from the vulva (external genital organs) to the cervix of the uterus.

vascular—pertaining to blood vessels.

vas deferens—a duct (tube) from the epididymis to the seminal vesicles for the transport of spermatozoa.

vasectomy—surgical removal of a portion of the vas deferens to induce infertility.

vasoconstriction—the diminution of the caliber of vessels, especially constriction of small arteries, which causes a decreased blood flow to an organ or body part.

vellus hair—the downy hair growing on the body during prepuberal years.

viropause—andropause.

vitiligo—condition characterized by destruction of melanocytes resulting in patches of depigmentation of the skin.

BIBLIOGRAPHY

Arver, S., A. S. Dobs, A. W. Meikle, R. P. Allen, S. W. Sanders, and N. A. Mazer. 1996, May. Improvement in sexual function in testosterone deficient men treated for 1 year with a permeation enhanced testosterone transdermal system. *J Urol* 155(5):1604–8.

Bancroft, J., and F. C. W. Wu. 1983. Changes in erectile responsiveness during androgen replacement therapy. *Arch Sex Behav* 12:59.

Bebb, R. A., B. D. Anawalt, R. B. Christensen, C. A. Paulsen, W. J. Bremner, and A. M. Matsumoto. 1996, February. Combined administration of levonorgestrel and testosterone induces more rapid and effective suppression of spermatogenesis than testosterone alone: a promising male contraceptive approach. *J Clin Endocrinol & Metab* 81(2):757–62.

Bennett, A. 1981. Medical research council working party on mild to moderate hypertension. *Lancet* 2:539.

Benson, G. 1994. *Endocrine factors related to impotence.* In *Impotence*, ed. A. H. Bennett. Philadelphia: Saunders.

Bhasin, S., R. S. Swerdloff, B. Steiner, M. A. Peterson, T. Meidores, M. Galmirini, M. R. Pandian, R. Goldberg, and

N. Berman. 1992, January. A biodegradable testosterone microcapsule formulation provides uniform eugonadal levels of testosterone (for 10 weeks in hypogonadal men.) *J Clin Endocrinol & Metab* 74(1):75–83.

Bhasin, S., T. W. Storer, N. Berman, C. Callegari, B. Clevenger, J. Phillips, T. J. Bunnell, R. Tricker, A. Shirazi, and R. Casaburi. 1996, July. The effects of supraphysiologic doses of testosterone on muscle size and strength in normal men. *N Eng J Med* 335(1):1–7.

Blouin, A. G., and G. S. Goldfield. 1995, September. Body image and steroid use in male body builders. *Int J Eating Disorders* 18(2):159–65.

Bolt, J. W., C. Evans, and V. R. Marshal. 1986. Sexual dysfunction after prostatectomy. *Br J Ural* 58:319.

Braunstein, G. D. 1994. *Testes.* In *Basic and clinical endocrinology,* 4th ed., ed. F. S. Greenspan, and J. D. Baxter. Norwalk, CT: Appleton and Lange.

Burk, J. P. 1994. *Impotence.* Philadelphia: Saunders.

Buyukgebiz, A. 1995. Treatment of constitutional delayed puberty with a combination of testosterone esters. *Hormone Research* 44 Suppl 3:32–4.

Carani, C., A. R. Granata, J. Bancroft, and P. Marrama. 1995. The effects of testosterone replacement on nocturnal penile tumescence and rigidity and erectile response to visual erotic stimuli in hypogonadal men. *Psychoneuroendocrinol* 20(7):743–53.

Carlstom, K., et al. 1992 September. Detection of testosterone administration by increased ratio between serum concentrations of testosterone and 17 alpha-hydroxyprogesterone. *Clin Chem* 38(9):1779–84.

Carrier, S., G. Brock, N. Kour, and T. F. Wand Lue. 1993. Pathophysiology of erectile dysfunction. 42:468–81.

Carter, J. N., J. E. Tyson, G. Tolis, et al. 1978. Prolactin-secreting tumors and hypogonadism in 22 men. *N Engl J Medications* 199:847.

Choi, P. Y., and H. G. Pape, Jr. 1994, March. Violence toward women and illicit androgenic-anabolic steroid use. *Annuals Clin Psychiatry* 6(1):21–5.

Cunningham, G. R., et al. 1989. *JAMA* 261:2525.

Davidson, C. S. 1996. *Physicians desk reference.* Montvale, NJ: Medical Economics.

Davis, S. R., P. McCloud, B. J. Strauss, and H. Burger. 1995, April. Testosterone enhances estradiol's effects on postmenopausal bone density and sexuality. *Maturitas* 21(3):227–36.

De Peceoli, B., F. Giada, A. Benettini, F. Sartori, and E. Piccalo. 1991, August. Anabolic steroid use in body builders: an echocardiographic study of left ventricle morphology and function. *Interp J Sports Med* 12(4):408–12.

Deyssig, R., and M. Weissel. 1993, April. Ingestion of androgenic-anabolic steroids induces mild thyroid impairment in the male body builders. *J Clin Endocrinol & Metab* 76(4):1069–71.

Drug evaluations. 1992, Fall. Chicago: American Medical Association.

Frankle, M. A., R. Eichberg, and S. B. Zachariah. 1988, August. Anabolic-androgenic steroids and a stroke in an athlete: case report. *Arch Phys Med & Rehab* 69(8):682–3.

Frishman, R. G. 1996 Oct. Hormone replacement therapy for men. *Harvard Health Letter* 21:6–8.

Fulow, W. L. 1985. Prevalence of impotence in the United States. *Med Aspects Hum Sex* 19:13.

Goh, H. H., D. F. Loke, and S. S. Ratnam. 1995, January. The impact of long-term testosterone replacement therapy on lipids and lipoprotein profiles in women. *Maturitas* 21(1):65–70.

Gomoa, A., et al. 1996, June. Tropical treatment of erectile dysfunction: a randomized double blind placebo controlled trial of cream containing aminopylline, isosorbide dinitrate, and co-dergocrine mesylate. *BMJ* 312:1512–5.

Greenspan, S. L., and N. M. Resnick. 1984. *Geriatric endocrinology*. In *Basic and clinical endocrinology*, 4th ed. Norwalk, CT: Appleton and Lange.

Guezennec, C. Y., J. P. Lafarge, V. A. Bricout, D. Merino, and B. Serrurier. 1995, August. Effect of competition stress on tests used to assess testosterone administration in athletes. *Int J Sports Med* 16(6):368–72.

Hargreave, T. B., and T. P. Stephensen. 1977. Potency and prostatectomy. *Br J Ural* 49:683.

Harman, J. G., and L. E. Limbird, eds. 1996. *Goodman and Gilman's pharmacological basis of therapeutics*, 9th ed. New York: McGraw-Hill.

Heaton, J. P. W., A. Morales, J. Owen, et al. 1990. Topical glyceryltrinitrate causes measurable penile arterial dilation in impotent men. *J Ural* 143:729.

Herbert, J. 1995. *Lancet* 345:1193.

Husten, L. 1995, February. Second thoughts about antioxidants. *Harvard Health Letter* 20:4–6.

Jensen, R. T., M. J. Collen, S. J. Pandol, et al. 1983. Cimetidine induced impotence and breast changes in patients with gastric hyper secretory states. *N Eng J Medications* 308:833.

Johnson, N. P. 1990, January. Was superman a supreme junky? The fallacy of anabolic steroids. *J So Carolina Med Assoc* 86(1):46–8.

Kalimi, M., and W. Regelson, eds. 1990. *The biologic role of dehydroepiandrosterone*. New York: de Gruyter.

Kedric, K. and C. Markland. 1975. The effects of pharmaco-
logic agents on ejaculation. *J Urol* 114:569.

Kicman, A. T., D. A. Cowan, L. Myhre, S. Nilsson, S. Tomten,
and H. Oftebro. 1994, November. Effect on sports
drug tests of ingesting meat from steroid (methen-
olone)-treated livestock. *Clin Chem* 40(11 Pt 1):
2084–7.

Kinsey, A. C., W. B. Pomroy, and C. E. Martin. 1979. *Sexual
behavior in the human male.* Philadelphia: Saunders.

Kornman, S. G., J. E. Moreley, A. D. Mooradion, et al. 1990.
Secondary hypogonadism in older men: its relationship
to impotence. *J Clin Endoc Metab* 71:963.

Lamb, D. R. 1994, January–February. Anabolic steroids in athletes: how well do they work and how dangerous are
they? *Am J Sports Med* 12(1):31–8.

Lane, J. R., and J. D. Connor. 1994, December. The influence
of endogenous and exogenous sex hormones in adolescents with attention to oral contraception and anabolic
steroids. *J Adoles Health* 14(8):630–4.

Laseter, J. T., and J. A. Russell. 1991 Jan. Anabolic steroid-
induced tendon pathology: a review of the literature.
Med & Sci in Sports & Ex 23(1):1–3.

Lehrman, S. 1995, January. Can the clock be slowed? *Harvard
Health Letter* 20(3):1–3.

Liao, S. 1996, October. Human prostate tumor growth in
athymic mice: inhibition by androgenic oral stimulation
of finasteride. *Proceedings Nat Acad Sci,* vol. 93.

Lue, T. F. 1990. Impotence: a patient goal-directed approach
to treatment. *World J Urol* 8:67–74.

Lukas, S. E. 1993, February. Current perspectives on anabolic-
androgenic steroid abuse. *Trends Pharmacol Sci* 14(2):
61–8.

Bibliography

Malone, D. A., Jr., and R. J. Dimeff. 1992, April. The use of fluoxetine in depression associated with anabolic steroid withdrawal: a case series. *J Clin Psychiatry* 53(4):130–2.

Margolis, A., P. Prieto, and L. Stein. 1971. Statistical summaries of 10,000 male cases using Afradexin in the treatment of impotence. *Curr The Res* 13:616.

Marin, P. 1995, November. Testosterone and regional fat distribution. *Obesity Res* 3 Suppl 4:609S–612S.

Marin, P., et al. 1992, December. The effects of testosterone treatment on body composition and metabolism of middle-aged obese men. *J Obes & Rel Metab Dis* 16(12):991–7.

Masters, W. M., and V. E. Johnson. 1966. *Human Sexual Response.* Boston: Little, Brown.

Matsumoto, A. M. 1994. *Endocrinol Metab Clin N Am* 23:857.

Meikle, A. W., et al. 1992 Mar. Enhanced transdermal delivery of testosterone across nonscrotal skin produces physiological concentrations of testosterone and its metabolites in hypogonadal men. *J Clin Endocrinol & Metab* 74(3):623–8.

Mendelson, J. D., J. Mendelson, and V. D. Patch. 1975. Plasma testosterone levels in heroin addiction and during methadone maintenance. *J Pharmacal Exp The* 192:211.

Mitchell, L. E., D. L. Spreaker, I. B. Borechi, T. Rice, P. M. Larkorzewski, and D. C. Rao. 1994. Evidence for an association between dehydroepiandrosterone sulfate and non-fatal, premature myocardial infarcts in males. Washington University, St. Louis; University of Cincinnati, Ohio, *Circulation* 89:89–93.

Mootman, T. J., and D. K. Montague. 1986. Routine endocrine screening in impotence. *Urol* 27:499.

Morales, A., B. Johnston, J. W. Heaton, and A. Clark. 1994, October. Oral androgens in the treatment of hypogonadal men. *J Urol* 152(4):1115–8.

Morales, A. J., et al. 1994. *J Clin Endocrinol Metab* 78:1360.

Morley, J. E., et al. 1993, February. Effects of testosterone replacement therapy in old hypogonadal males: a preliminary study. *J Am Ger Soc* 41(2):149–52.

Murdock, M. I. 1993. Prostaglandin E-1: a problem-free medication. *Impotence Worldwide* 9(4):2–3.

Muto, M., H. Furumoto, A. Ohmura, and C. Asagami. 1995, October. Successful treatment of vitiligo with a sex steroid–thyroid hormone mixture. *J Dermatol* 22(10): 770–2.

National hospital discharge survey, 1985. 1989. National Center for Health Statistics, Department of Health and Human Services. 87:1751.

Ozata, M., M. Yildirimakaya, M. Bulur, K. Yilmaz, E. Bolu, A. Corakci, and M. A. Gundogan. 1996, September. Effects of gonadrotropin and testosterone treatments on Lipoprotein(a), high density lipoprotein particles, and other lipoprotein levels in male hypogonadism. *J Clin Endocrinol & Metab* 81(9):3372–8.

Ozhar, J., D. Meiroz, and B. Moaz. 1976. Factors influencing sexual activity after prostatectomy: a prospective study. *J Ural* 116:332.

Parcerelli, J. H., and B. A. Sandler. 1995, November. Narcissism and empathy in steroid users. *J Psychiatry* 152(11):1672–4.

Parrott, A. C., P. Y. Choi, and M. Davies. 1994, September. Anabolic steroid use by amateur athletes: effects upon psychological mood states. *J Sports Med & Phys Fitness* 34(3):292–8.

Perryman, R. L., and M. O. Thorner. 1981. The effects of hyperprolactinemia on sexual and reproductive function in men. *J Andral* 5:233.

Pope, H. J., Jr., and D. L. Katz. 1994, May. Psychiatric and medical effects of anabolic-androgenic steroid use. A controlled study of 160 athletes. *Arch Gen Psychiatry* 51(5):375–82.

Pravone-Mocaluso, M., V. Serreta, G. Daricello, and C. Pavone. 1990. Is there a role for pure antiandrogens in the treatment of advanced prostatic cancer? *Prog Clin Biol Res* 350:149.

Rabkin, J. G., R. Rabkin, and G. Wagner. 1995, January. Testosterone replacement therapy in HIV illness. *Gen Hosp Psychiatry* 17(1):37–42.

Rako, S. 1996. *The Hormone of Desire.* New York: Harmony Books.

Regelson, W. 1996. *The Superhormone Promise.* New York: Simon and Schuster.

Reid, K., D. H. Surridge, A. Morales, et al. 1987. Double-blind trials of yohimbine in treatment of psychogenic impotence. *Lancet* 2:421.

Rubin, H. B. and D. E. Hanson. 1979. *Effects of drugs on male sexual function.* In *Advances in Behavioral Pharmacology,* ed. T. Thompson and P. B. Days. New York: Academic Press.

Savage, M. W., P. Reed, S. L. Orrman-Rossiter, C. Weinkove, and D. C. Anderson. 1992, June. Acute intermittent porphyria treated by testosterone implant. *Postgrad Med J* 68(800):479–81.

Savvas, M., J. Bishop, G. Laurent, N. Watson, and J. Studd. 1993, February. Type III collagen content in the skin of postmenopausal women receiving oestradiol and testosterone implants. *Br J Obstet & Gynaecol* 100(2):154–6.

Savvas, M., J. W. Studl, S. Norman, A. T. Leather, T. J. Garnett, and J. Fogellman. 1992, September. Increase in bone mass after one year of percutaneous oestradiol and testosterone implants in post-menopausal women who have previously received long-term oral oestrogens. *Brit J Obstet & Gynaecol* 99(9):757–60.

Shaban, S. T. 1991. *Treatment of abnormalities of ejaculation.* In *Infertility in the male,* 2d ed., ed. L. I. Lipschutz and S. S. Howards. St. Louis: Mosby Year Book.

Shabsingh, R., I. J. Fishman, and Z. B. Scot. 1988. Evaluation of erectile impotence. *Urol* 32–83.

Shapiro, T., and M. Herzig. 1988. Normal growth and development. In *The American Psychiatric Press textbook of psychiatry.* Washington, D.C.: American Psychiatric Press.

Sideri, M., M. Origoni, L. Spinaci, and A. Ferrari. 1994, July. Topical testosterone in the treatment of vulvar lichen sclerosus. *Int J Gynaecol & Obstet* 46(1):53–6.

Slab, A. K., J. J. Van der Werff ten Bosch, E. V. Van Hall, F. H. deJong, W. C. Weijmar Schultz, and F. A. Eiklboon. 1993, Fall. Psychosocial functioning in women with complete testicular feminization: is androgen replacement therapy preferable to estrogen? *J Sex & Marital Ther* 19(3):201–9.

Stanley, A., and M. Ward. 1994, January. Anabolic steroids, F. H. deJong, W. C. Weijmar Schultz, and F *Med Sci & Law.* 34(1):82–3.

Tenover, J. S. 1992, October. Effects of testosterone supplementation in the aging male. *J Clin Endocrinol & Metab* 75(4):1092–8.

"Testosterone for the Aging Male." 1996, 10 August. Continuing Education Seminar, Division of Endocrinology, Diabetes and Clinical Nutrition, Oregon Health Sciences University.

Vallery-Masson, J., A. J. Valleron, and J. Poitrenaud. 1981. Factors related to sexual intercourse frequency in a group of French pre-retirement managers. *Aging* 10:53–9.

Bibliography

Van Goozen, S. H., P. T. Cohen-Kettenis, L. J. Gooren, N. H. Frijda, and N. E. Van de Poll. 1994, October. Activating effects of androgens on cognitive performance: casual evidence in a group of female-to-male transsexuals. *Neuropsychologia* 32(10):1153–7.

van Vollenhoven, R. F., et al. 1995. *Arthritis Rheum* 38:1826.

Villareal, D. T., and J. E. Morley. 1994, June. Trophic factors in aging: should older people receive hormonal replacement therapy? *Drugs & Aging* 4(6):492–509.

Wasserman, M. D., C. P. Pollack, and A. J. Spielman. 1980. Impaired nocturnal erections and impotence following transurethral prostatectomy. *Urol* 15:552.

Welder, A. A., and R. B. Melchert. 1993, April. Cardiotonic effects of cocaine and anabolic-androgenic steroids on athletes. [Review] *J Pharmacolog & Toxicolog Meth* 29(2):61–8.

Witherington, R. 1985. The Osborn Erecaid system in the management of erectile impotence. *J Urol* 33A:306.

Yen, S. S. C., et al. 1995. *Ann NY Acad Sci.* 774:128.

Yendt, E. R., G. F. Gray, and D. A. Garcia. 1970. The use of thiazides in prevention of renal calculi. *Con Med Assoc J* 102:614.

Zarren, H. S., and P. M. Block. 1995. Unilateral gynecomastia and impotence during low dose spirolactone administration in men. *Mil Med* 140:417.

INDEX

Index

Index

testosterone
  influence of testosterone on
    growth and development,
    180–182
  life cycle of testosterone,
    179–180
  medical conditions affecting
    testosterone, 195–199
  production of testosterone in
    the body, 177–178
endothelium, 194
epitestosterone, 120
erections
  blood flow and cartilage changes,
    19–20, 153
  difficulties having, 4, 21–22
  necessity for orgasm, 21
  testosterone and, 22–23
ergot, 147
estradiol, 177
estrogen and other female hormones,
  39, 172, 177. *See also* women's
  health
ethics, medical, 147–149

F
female sexuality. *See* gender differences; women's health
Fenfluramine, 109
5–alpha-reductase inhibitor, 170, 173
fluoxymesterone (Halotestin), 125
Flutamide, 170
free radicals, 39–40
Freud, Sigmund, 13–14
FSH (follicle stimulating hormone),
  35, 178

G
gender differences. *See also* women's
  health
  cognitive, 141
  desire for relationships, 16–17
  hormone deficiencies in men and
    women (comparison),
    201–204

libido by age of men and women
  (comparison), 17
need for sexual gratification,
  14–15
response to members of the opposite sex, 15
sex hormones by age of men and
  women (comparison), 33
glyceryltrinitrate, 109
gonadotropic hormones, 122
gonads, 176

H
hGH (human growth hormone),
  7, 41
hormones, 175–176. *See also*
  endocrine system; testosterone
  testosterone and other male hormones, 177
hyperplasia, 114
hyperprolactinemia, 19
hypogonadism, 34, 59, 198
hypothalamus, 176–177
hypothyroidism, 132

I
implants, prosthetic 110–112
impotence. *See* sexual dysfunction
injections, penile, 110–112
introitus, 20
intromission, 20
isosorbide, 147

J
Jung, Carl, 14

K
Klinefelter's syndrome, 196

L
L-dopa, 109
Leydig cells, 35, 164
LH (luteinizing hormone), 35, 178
libido, 12–19

Index

Index

osteoporosis and, 142–143

production in the body (testes, adrenal glands), 152, 178

production of synthetic hormone, 59

testosterone deficiency. *See also* medical factors affecting testosterone levels

a medical view of, 36–37

and andropause, 90–96

and sexuality, 48–50

case history, 73–84

changes in memory and cognition, 55

depression resulting from, 49, 53–54

diagnosis of, 4–5, 94–95

duration, 94

external vs. internal testosterone sources, 6

onset, 92

osteoporosis, 50–53, 142–143

prognosis, 96

symptoms of 3–5, 92–93

treatment of, 95–96

vigor and aggressiveness, 47

testosterone replacement therapy (TRT), 6, 36, 52–59, 106–108. *See also* creams

benefits of, 8–9, 60–61, 62–63

body fat, 63

bone strength, 63

diabetes, 63

heart disease, 63

muscle mass and strength, 62

sexual functioning, 61–62

blood tests, 69

cost, 156

length of treatment, 68–69, 156

methods of administration, 63–67

injections, 64–65

patches, 65–67

tablets, 64

prognosis, 72

side effects, 69–72

allergic reactions, 70

long-term side effects, 70

therapeutic (or diagnostic) trials, 133

thromboses (clots), 123

thymus, 176

thyroid and thyroid conditions, 176

hyperthyroidism, 48

thyrotoxosis, 51

Turner's syndrome, 196

TURP (transurethral resection prostatectomy), 115

U

urinary difficulties. *See* prostate

V

Viagro, 144

viropause, 86. *See* andropause (male menopause)

vitamins, 40

W

women's health

estrogen, 39 172

and cognition, 141–142

and estradiol, estrone, and estiol, 177

combined with testosterone, 132–133

receptors, 55

Hormone of Desire (Susan Roko), 133

menopause, 131–133

osteoporosis, 52

testosterone therapy for women, 129–137

for menopause, 132–134

for other conditions, 134–135

side effects, 136–137, 154

The Complete Prostate Book

Every Man's Guide

Lee Belshin, M.S.

U.S. $14.95
Can. $19.95
ISBN 0-7615-0447-8
paperback / 240 pages

Over half of all men will experience prostate problems during their lifetimes. But most men are only vaguely aware of the various disorders, their treatments, and aftereffects. With *The Complete Prostate Book*, you will discover how prostate cancer, prostate enlargement, and related health problems can be overcome. In simple and friendly terms, author and public health educator Lee Belshin explains everything you need to know about prostate conditions, from what to expect when you visit the doctor's office to an overview of possible treatments. He also shares encouraging stories from his own and other men's battles against prostate problems.

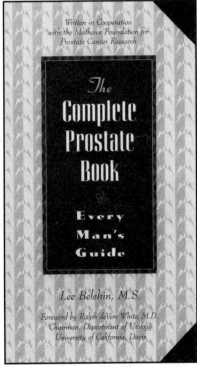

Visit us online at www.primapublishing.com

To Order Books

Please send me the following items:

Quantity	Title	Unit Price	Total
_____	<u>The Complete Prostate Book</u>	$ <u>14.95</u>	$ _____
_____	_____	$ _____	$ _____
_____	_____	$ _____	$ _____
_____	_____	$ _____	$ _____
_____	_____	$ _____	$ _____

*Shipping and Handling depend on Subtotal.

Subtotal	Shipping/Handling
$0.00–$14.99	$3.00
$15.00–$29.99	$4.00
$30.00–$49.99	$6.00
$50.00–$99.99	$10.00
$100.00–$199.99	$13.50
$200.00+	Call for Quote

Foreign and all Priority Request orders:
Call Order Entry department
for price quote at 916-632-4400

This chart represents the total retail price of books only (before applicable discounts are taken).

Subtotal $ _____

Deduct 10% when ordering 3-5 books $ _____

7.25% Sales Tax (CA only) $ _____

8.25% Sales Tax (TN only) $ _____

5.0% Sales Tax (MD and IN only) $ _____

7.0% G.S.T. Tax (Canada only) $ _____

Shipping and Handling* $ _____

Total Order $ _____

By Telephone: With MC or Visa, call 800-632-8676 or 916-632-4400.
Mon–Fri, 8:30-4:30.

WWW: http://www.primapublishing.com

By Internet E-mail: sales@primapub.com

By Mail: Just fill out the information below and send with your remittance to:

Prima Publishing
P.O. Box 1260BK
Rocklin, CA 95677

My name is _____

I live at _____

City _____ State _____ ZIP _____

MC/Visa#_____ Exp. _____

Check/money order enclosed for $ _____ Payable to Prima Publishing

Daytime telephone _____

Signature _____